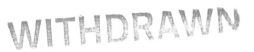

The Respiratory System at a Glance

JEREMY P.T. WARD

PhD
Professor of Respiratory Cell Physiology
Department of Respiratory Medicine and Allergy
Guy's, King's and St Thomas' School of Medicine
King's College London
London, UK

JANE WARD

MBChB, PhD
Senior Lecturer
Applied Biomedical Sciences Research
Guy's, King's and St Thomas' School of Biomedical Sciences
King's College London
London, UK

CHARLES M. WIENER

MD
Associate Professor of Medicine and Physiology
Department of Medicine
Johns Hopkins School of Medicine
Baltimore MD, USA

RICHARD M. LEACH

FRCP, MD
Honorary Senior Lecturer
Department of Respiratory Medicine and Allergy, and Intensive Care
Guy's, King's and St Thomas' School of Medicine
St Thomas' Hospital
London, UK

Blackwell
Science

© 2002 by Blackwell Science Ltd
a Blackwell Publishing company
Blackwell Science, Inc., 350 Main Street, Malden, Massachusetts 02148-5018, USA
Blackwell Science Ltd, Osney Mead, Oxford OX2 0EL, UK
Blackwell Science Asia Pty Ltd, 550 Swanston Street, Carlton, Victoria 3053, Australia
Blackwell Wissenschafts Verlag, Kurfürstendamm 57, 10707 Berlin, Germany

First published 2002

Library of Congress Cataloging-in-Publication Data

The respiratory system at a glance / Jeremy Ward . . . [et al.].
        p. ; cm.
Includes index.
    ISBN 0-632-06447-1 (pbk.)
    1. Respiratory organs — Diseases.
    [DNLM: 1.   Respiratory Physiology.   2.   Respiratory
System — physiopathology. WF 102 R437 2002]   I.   Ward, Jeremy P.T.
RC731 .R493 2002
616.2 — dc21

                                                                    2001008081

ISBN 0-632-06447-1

A catalogue record for this title is available from the British Library

Set in 9/11.5 Times by SNP Best-set Typesetter Ltd., Hong Kong
Printed and bound in the United Kingdom by MPG Books Ltd, Bodmin, Cornwall

Commissioning Editor: Fiona Goodgame
Managing Editor: Geraldine Jeffers
Editorial Assistant: Vicky Pinder
Production Editor: Lorna Hind
Production Controller: Kate Charman

For further information on Blackwell Science, visit our website:
www.blackwell-science.com

Contents

Preface

Over the last few years the medical curriculum has become increasingly vertically integrated, with a much greater use of clinical examples and cases for teaching the underlying science, and basic science concepts to help understanding of the pathophysiology and treatment of disease. *The Respiratory System at a Glance*, like its sibling, *The Cardiovascular System at a Glance*, has been written to take account of this trend, and integrate core aspects of basic science, pathophysiology and treatment into a single, easy to use revision aid. As such, it should be useful to medical students throughout their training, and also to other healthcare professions, including nursing.

As with other volumes in the *At a Glance* series, it is based around a two-page spread for each main topic, with figures and text complementing each other to give an overview of a topic at a glance. Case studies based on some of the most commonly encountered conditions are also provided, and can be used for both basic science and clinical study. Although primarily designed for revision, the book covers all the core elements of the respiratory system and its major diseases, and as such could be used as a main text in the first couple of years of the course. It is, however, advised that additional reference to more detailed textbooks will aid deeper and wider understanding of the subject. This is particularly the case for the pathophysiological chapters, as a book of this length cannot hope to provide a complete guide to clinical practice.

However carefully written, first editions always contain some errors and omissions, and these are entirely our responsibility, and not those of our colleagues who have kindly advised us and commented on the contents. We would also like to thank all the staff at Blackwell Publishing who have assisted us in producing this volume, particularly Fiona Goodgame and Anita Lane who cajoled us into meeting at least one deadline.

Jeremy Ward
Jane Ward
Charles Wiener
Richard Leach

Units, symbols and abbreviations

Units

The medical profession and scientific community generally use SI (Système International) units.

Pressure conversion: SI unit of pressure: 1 pascal (Pa) = $1 N \cdot m^{-2}$. As this is small, in medicine the kPa ($=10^3$ Pa) is more commonly used. Note that millimetres of mercury (mmHg) are still the commonest unit for expressing arterial and venous blood pressures, and low pressures—e.g. central venous pressure and intrapleural pressure—are sometimes expressed as centimeters of H_2O (cm H_2O). Blood gas partial pressures are reported by some laboratories in kPa and by some in mmHg, so you need to be familiar with both systems.

1 kPa = 7.5 mmHg = 10.2 cmH_2O
1 mmHg = 1 torr = 0.133 kPa = 1.36 cmH_2O
1 cmH_2O = 0.098 kPa = 0.74 mmHg
1 standard atmosphere ($\approx$1 bar) = 101.3 kPa = 760 mmHg = 1033 cm H_2O

Contents are still commonly expressed per 100 mL (dL^{-1}), and these need to be multiplied by 10 to give the more standard SI unit per litre. Contents are also increasingly being expressed as mmol$\cdot$L^{-1}.

For haemoglobin: 1 g$\cdot$dL^{-1} = 10 g$\cdot$L^{-1} = 0.062 mmol$\cdot$L^{-1}

For ideal gases (including oxygen and nitrogen): 1 mmol = 22.4 mL standard temperature and pressure dry (STPD; see Chapter 4)

For non-ideal gases, such as nitrous oxide and carbon dioxide: 1 mmol = 22.25 mL STPD

Symbols

Symbols used in respiratory and cardiovascular physiology are given in Fig. 4 (Chapter 4)

Typical inspired, alveolar and blood gas values in healthy young adults are shown in the table below. Ranges are given for arterial blood gas values. Mean arterial P_{O_2} falls with age, and by 60 years is about 11 kPa/82 mmHg. Typical values for lung volumes and other lung function tests are given in the appropriate chapters. Ranges for many values are affected by age, sex and height, as well as by the method of measurement, and hence it is necessary to refer to appropriate nomograms.

Inspired P_{O_2} (dry, sea level)	21 kPa	159 mmHg
Alveolar P_{O_2}	13.3 kPa	100 mmHg
Arterial P_{O_2}	12.5 (11.2–13.9) kPa	94 (84–104) mmHg
A–a P_{O_2} gradient	<2 kPa	<15 mmHg (greater in elderly)
Oxygen saturation	>97%	
Oxygen content	20 mL$\cdot$dL^{-1}	
Inspired P_{CO_2}	0.03 kPa	0.2 mmHg
Alveolar P_{CO_2}	5.3 (4.7–6.1) kPa	40 (35–45) mmHg
Arterial P_{CO_2}	5.3 (4.7–6.1) kPa	40 (35–45) mmHg
Arterial CO_2 content	48 mL$\cdot$dL^{-1}	
Arterial [H$^+$] / pH	36–44 nmol$\cdot$L^{-1} / 7.44–7.36	
Resting mixed venous P_{O_2}	5.3 kPa	40 mmHg
Resting mixed venous O_2 content	15 mL$\cdot$dL^{-1}	
Resting oxygen saturation	75%	
Resting mixed venous P_{CO_2}	6.1 kPa	46 mmHg
Resting mixed venous CO_2 content	52 mL$\cdot$dL^{-1}	
Arterial [HCO$_3^-$]	24 (21–27) mM	

Abbreviations used in this book

Abbreviation	Definition
A–a gradient	(A–a P_{O_2}) gradient, the difference between ideal alveolar and arterial P_{O_2}
AAT	α_1-antitrypsin
AFB	acid-fast bacillus
AHI	apnoea plus hypopnoea index
AIDS	acquired immune deficiency syndrome
AIP	acute interstitial pneumonia/pneumonitis (Hamman–Rich syndrome)
ALI	acute lung injury
ANA	anti-nuclear antibody
ANCA	antineutrophil cytoplasmic antibody
ARDS	acute (formerly adult) respiratory distress syndrome
ATPS	ambient temperature and pressure saturated
BAL	bronchoalveolar lavage
BALT	bronchus associated lymphoid tissue
BCG	bacille Calmette–Guérin
BiPAP	biphasic positive pressure ventilation
BTPS	body temperature and pressure saturated
CA	carbonic anhydrase
cAMP	cyclic adenosine monophosphate
CCF	congestive cardiac failure
CF	cystic fibrosis
CFA	cryptogenic fibrosing alveolitis
CFTR	cystic fibrosis transmembrane conductance regulator
C_L	lung compliance = $\Delta V/\Delta P$, where P = alveolar–intrapleural pressure
CMV	controlled mechanical ventilation
CMV	cytomegalovirus
CNS	central nervous system
COAD	chronic obstructive airway disease (synonymous with COPD, COLD)
COLD	chronic obstructive lung disease (synonymous with COAD, COPD)
COPD	chronic obstructive pulmonary disease (synonymous with COAD, COLD)
COX	cyclooxygenase
CPAP	continuous positive airway pressure
CREST	calcinosis, Raynaud's phenomenon, esophageal involvement, sclerodactyly, and telangiectasi
CSA	central sleep apnoea
CSB	Cheyne–Stokes breathing
CSF	cerebrospinal fluid
CT	computed tomography
CWP	coal workers' pneumoconiosis
CXR	chest X-ray
DIP	desquamative interstitial pneumonia
D_LCO	diffusing capacity of the lungs for carbon monoxide
D_Lg	diffusing capacity of the lungs for gas
D_LO_2	diffusing capacity of the lungs for oxygen
D_TCO	carbon monoxide transfer factor (alternative name for D_LCO)
DVT	deep vein thrombosis
EBV	Epstein–Barr virus
ECG	electrocardiogram
ECMO	extracorporeal membrane oxygenation
ECP	eosinophil cationic protein
EEG	electroencephalogram
EGF	epidermal growth factor
ELISA	enzyme-linked immunoassay
EMG	electromyogram
EOG	electrooculogram
ERV	expiratory reserve volume
ESR	erythrocyte sedimentation rate
FDG	fluorodeoxyglucose
FDG PET	fluorodeoxyglucose positron emission tomography
FEF_{25-75}	mean forced expiratory flow over middle 50% of forced vital capacity
FEV_1	forced expiratory volume in 1 second
FEV_1/FVC	FEV_1 expressed as a fraction, or more usually a percentage of FVC
FGF	fibroblast growth factor
FRC	functional residual capacity
FVC	forced vital capacity
GBM	glomerular basement membrane
GM-CSF	granulocyte macrophage colony stimulating factor
GU	genitourinary
HAART	highly active antiretroviral therapy
HIV	human immunodeficiency virus
HRCT	high-resolution computed tomography
IFN-γ	interferon-γ
Ig	immunoglobulin, e.g. IgA, IgE, IgG, IgM
IL	interleukin, e.g. IL-10
ILD	interstitial lung disease
INPV	intermittent negative pressure ventilation
IPF	idiopathic pulmonary fibrosis (synonymous with CFA)
IPPV	intermittent positive pressure breathing
IRV	inspiratory reserve volume
IVC	inferior vena cava
K_{CO}	D_LCO divided by alveolar volume or Krough coefficient
KS	Kaposi's sarcoma
LDH	lactate dehydrogenase
LG	lymphomatoid granulomatosis
LIP	lymphocytic interstitial pneumonia
LMWH	low molecular weight heparin
LT	leukotriene, e.g. LTC_4
LV	left ventricle, left ventricular
MAC	*Mycobacterium avium* complex
MBP	major basic protein
MI	myocardial infarction
MIE	meconium ileus equivalent
MMV	mandatory minute ventilation
MOF	multiorgan failure
MPA	microscopic polyangiitis
MTB	mycobacterium tuberculosis
MVV	maximal voluntary ventilation
NANC	non-adrenergic, non-cholinergic (nerves)
NHL	non-Hodgkin's lymphoma
NIPPV	non-invasive positive pressure ventilation
NRDS	neonatal respiratory distress syndrome
NREM	non-rapid eye movement
NSAID	non-steroidal anti-inflammatory drug
NSC	non-small cell
NSIP	non-specific interstitial pneumonia
OSA	obstructive sleep apnoea
P_{50}	partial pressure at which haemoglobin is 50% saturated with O_2
P_A	alveolar pressure
PA	posterior–anterior
PA	pulmonary arterial
P_ACO	partial pressure of carbon monoxide in the alveoli
P_aCO_2	partial pressure of carbon dioxide in the blood
P_ACO_2	partial pressure of CO_2 in the alveoli
PAF	platelet-activating factor
PAN	polyarteritis nodosa
P_aO_2	partial pressure of oxygen in the arterial blood
PAV	pulmonary arterial vasculopathy (formerly primary pulmonary hypertension)

P_c	capillary pressure		RV	residual volume
PCP	*Pneumocystis carinii* pneumonia		RVD	restrictive ventilatory defect
$PD_{20}FEV_1$	provocative dose (eg. of histamine or methacholine) that induces a 20% fall in FEV_1		SC	small cell
			SIADH	syndrome of inappropriate secretion of anti-diuretic hormone
PE	pulmonary embolus		SIMV	synchronized intermittent mandatory ventilation
PEEP	positive end-expiratory pressure		SLE	systemic lupus erythematosus
PEFR	peak expiratory flow rate		So_2	oxygen saturation (oxygen content/oxygen capacity)
PET	positron emission tomography		STPD	standard temperature and pressure dry
Pg	prostaglandin, e.g. PgD_2		SV	spontaneous ventilation
pK_A	log of dissociation constant K_A		TB	tuberculosis
PM/DM	polymyositis/dermatomyositis		TGFβ	transforming growth factor β
PMF	progressive massive fibrosis		TLC	total lung capacity
PMI	point of maximal impulse (also known as Apex beat)		TNM	tumour, node and metastasis
PPD	purified protein derivative		UFH	unfractionated heparin
PSP	primary spontaneous pneumothorax		UIP	usual interstitial pneumonia
RAD	right axis deviation (electrocardiography)		V_A/Q	ventilation–perfusion ratio; (alveolar ventilation/blood flow in a lung region)
RANTES	regulated on activation normal T cell expressed and secreted		VC	vital capacity
RAW	airway resistance (mouth–alveolar pressure/airflow)		V_T	tidal volume
RBBB	right bundle branch block		WBC	white blood cell
RBC	red blood cell		WG	Wegener's granulomatosis
REM	rapid eye movement			

1 Structure of the respiratory system: lungs, airways and dead space

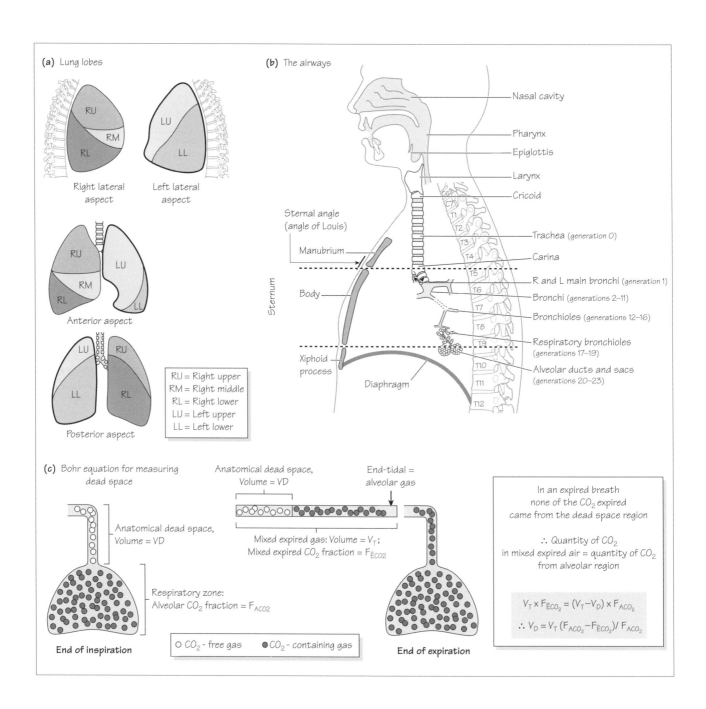

(a) Lung lobes

Right lateral aspect   Left lateral aspect

Anterior aspect

Posterior aspect

RU = Right upper
RM = Right middle
RL = Right lower
LU = Left upper
LL = Left lower

(b) The airways

Nasal cavity
Pharynx
Epiglottis
Larynx
Cricoid
Sternal angle (angle of Louis)
Manubrium
Body
Xiphoid process
Sternum
Trachea (generation 0)
Carina
R and L main bronchi (generation 1)
Bronchi (generations 2–11)
Bronchioles (generations 12–16)
Respiratory bronchioles (generations 17–19)
Alveolar ducts and sacs (generations 20–23)
Diaphragm

(c) Bohr equation for measuring dead space

Anatomical dead space, Volume = VD

End-tidal = alveolar gas

Anatomical dead space, Volume = VD

Mixed expired gas: Volume = V_T; Mixed expired CO_2 fraction = $F_{\bar{E}CO_2}$

Respiratory zone: Alveolar CO_2 fraction = F_{ACO_2}

End of inspiration

○ CO_2 - free gas   ● CO_2 - containing gas

End of expiration

In an expired breath none of the CO_2 expired came from the dead space region

∴ Quantity of CO_2 in mixed expired air = quantity of CO_2 from alveolar region

$$V_T \times F_{\bar{E}CO_2} = (V_T - V_D) \times F_{ACO_2}$$

$$\therefore V_D = V_T (F_{ACO_2} - F_{\bar{E}CO_2}) / F_{ACO_2}$$

Lungs

The respiratory system consists of a pair of **lungs** within the **thoracic cage** (Chapter 2). Its main function is gas exchange, but other roles include speech, filtration of microthrombi arriving from systemic veins and metabolic activities such as conversion of angiotensin I to angiotensin II and removal or deactivation of serotonin, bradykinin, norepinephrine, acetylcholine and drugs such as propranolol and chlorpromazine.

The **right lung** is divided by **transverse and oblique fissures** into three lobes: upper, middle and lower. The **left lung** has an **oblique fissure** and two lobes (Fig. 1a). Vessels, nerves and lymphatics enter the lungs on their medial surfaces at the lung root or **hilum**. Each lobe is divided into a number of wedge-shaped **bronchopulmonary segments** with their apices at the hilum and bases at the lung surface. Each bronchopulmonary segment is supplied by its own segmental bronchus, artery and vein and can be removed surgically with little bleeding or air leakage from the remaining lung.

The **pulmonary nerve plexus** lies behind each hilum, receiving fibres from both **vagi** and the 2nd to 4th thoracic **ganglia** of the **sympathetic trunk**. Each vagus contains sensory afferents from lungs and airways and bronchoconstrictor and secretomotor efferents. Sympathetic fibres are bronchodilator.

Each lung is lined by a thin membrane, the **visceral pleura**, which is continuous with the **parietal pleura**, lining the chest wall, diaphragm, pericardium and mediastinum. The space between the parietal and visceral layers is tiny in health and lubricated with pleural fluid. The right and left pleural cavities are separate and each extends as the **costodiaphragmatic recess** below the lungs even during full inspiration. The parietal pleura is segmentally innervated by **intercostal nerves** and by the **phrenic nerve**, and so pain from pleural inflammation (**pleurisy**) is often referred to the chest wall or shoulder tip. The visceral pleura lacks sensory innervation.

Lymph channels are absent in alveolar walls, but accompany small blood vessels conveying lymph towards the hilar **bronchopulmonary nodes** and from there to **tracheobronchial nodes** at the tracheal bifurcation. Some lymph from the lower lobe drains to the **posterior mediastinal nodes**.

The **upper respiratory tract** consists of the nose, pharynx and larynx. The **lower respiratory tract** (Fig. 1b) starts with the trachea at the lower border of the **cricoid cartilage**, level with the 6th cervical vertebra (C6). It bifurcates into **right and left main bronchi** at the level of the **sternal angle** and T4/5 (lower when upright and in inspiration). The right main bronchus is wider, shorter and more vertical than the left, so inhaled foreign bodies enter it more easily.

Airways

The airways divide repeatedly, with each successive **generation** approximately doubling in number. The **trachea** and **main bronchi** have U-shaped cartilage linked posteriorly by smooth muscle. Lobar bronchi supply the three right and two left lung lobes and divide to give **segmental bronchi** (generations 3 and 4). The total cross-sectional area of each generation is minimum here, after which it rises rapidly, as increased numbers more than make up for their reduced size. Generations 5–11 are small bronchi, the smallest being 1 mm in diameter. The lobar, segmental and small bronchi are supported by irregular plates of cartilage, with bronchial smooth muscle forming helical bands. **Bronchioles** start at about generation 12 and from this point on cartilage is absent. These airways are embedded in lung tissue, which holds them open like tent guy ropes. The **terminal bronchioles** (generation 16) lead to **respiratory bronchioles**, the first generation to have alveoli (Chapter 5) in their walls. These lead to **alveolar ducts** and **alveolar sacs** (generation 23), whose walls are entirely composed of **alveoli**.

The bronchi and airways down to the terminal bronchioles receive nutrition from the **bronchial arteries** arising from the descending aorta. The respiratory bronchioles, alveolar ducts and sacs are supplied by the **pulmonary circulation** (Chapter 13). The respiratory epithelium is discussed in Chapter 16.

Dead space

The upper respiratory tract and airways as far as the terminal bronchioles do not take part in gas exchange. These **conducting airways** form the **anatomical dead space** (V_D), whose volume is normally about 150 mL. These airways have an air-conditioning function, warming, filtering and humidifying inspired air.

Alveoli that have lost their blood supply—for example because of a **pulmonary embolus**—no longer take part in gas exchange and form **alveolar dead space**. The sum of the anatomical and alveolar dead space is known as the **physiological dead space**, ventilation of which is wasted in terms of gas exchange. In health, all alveoli take part in gas exchange, so physiological dead space equals anatomical dead space.

The volume of a breath or **tidal volume** (V_T), is about 500 mL at rest. Resting **respiratory frequency** (f) is about 15 breaths/min, so the volume entering the lungs each minute, the **minute ventilation**, is about 7500 mL/min ($= 500 \times 15$) at rest. **Alveolar ventilation** (V_A) is the volume taking part in gas exchange each minute. At rest, dead space volume = 150 mL and alveolar ventilation is 5250 mL/min ($= (500 - 150) \times 15$).

The **Bohr method** for measuring anatomical dead space is based on the principle that the degree to which dead space gas (0% CO_2) dilutes alveolar gas (about 5% CO_2) to give mixed expired gas (about 3.5%) depends on its volume (Fig. 1c). **Alveolar gas** can be sampled at the end of the breath as **end-tidal gas**. The Bohr equation can be modified to measure physiological dead space by using arterial P_{CO_2} to estimate the CO_2 in the gas-exchanging or **ideal alveoli**.

2 The thoracic cage and respiratory muscles

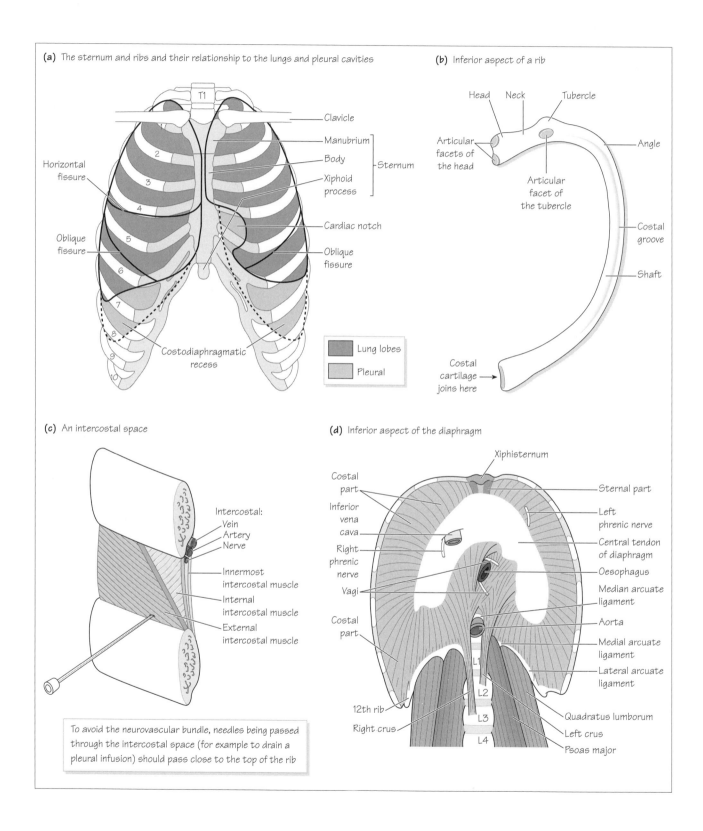

(a) The sternum and ribs and their relationship to the lungs and pleural cavities

T1

Clavicle

Manubrium

Body

Xiphoid process

— Sternum

Cardiac notch

Oblique fissure

Horizontal fissure

Oblique fissure

Costodiaphragmatic recess

Lung lobes

Pleural

(b) Inferior aspect of a rib

Head Neck Tubercle

Articular facets of the head

Articular facet of the tubercle

Angle

Costal groove

Shaft

Costal cartilage joins here

(c) An intercostal space

Intercostal:
Vein
Artery
Nerve

Innermost intercostal muscle

Internal intercostal muscle

External intercostal muscle

To avoid the neurovascular bundle, needles being passed through the intercostal space (for example to drain a pleural infusion) should pass close to the top of the rib

(d) Inferior aspect of the diaphragm

Xiphisternum

Sternal part

Left phrenic nerve

Central tendon of diaphragm

Oesophagus

Median arcuate ligament

Aorta

Medial arcuate ligament

Lateral arcuate ligament

Quadratus lumborum

Left crus

Psoas major

Costal part

Inferior vena cava

Right phrenic nerve

Vagi

Costal part

12th rib

Right crus

L1

L2

L3

L4

Thoracic cage

The **thoracic cage** is composed of the **sternum, ribs, intercostal spaces** and **thoracic vertebral column**, with the **diaphragm** dividing the thorax from the abdomen.

The dagger-shaped **sternum** has three parts. The **manubrium**, with which the first and upper parts of the second costal cartilage and the clavicle articulate (Fig. 2a), lies at the level of the third and fourth thoracic vertebrae (Fig. 2b). The lower parts of the second and third to seventh ribs articulate with the **body of the sternum** (level with T5–T8). The angle between the manubrium and body at the cartilaginous **manubriosternal joint** forms the **sternal angle (angle of Louis)** and this is a useful anatomical reference point. The small **xiphoid process** (xiphisternum) usually remains cartilaginous well into adult life.

The first seven (**true or vertebrosternal**) of the 12 pairs of ribs are connected to the sternum by their costal cartilages. The hyaline cartilages of the eighth, ninth and tenth (**vertebrochondral**) ribs articulate with the cartilage above, and the eleventh and twelfth are free (**floating or vertebral ribs**). A typical rib (Fig. 2b) has a **head** with two **facets** for articulation with the corresponding vertebra, the intervertebral disc and the vertebra above. The rib also articulates at the **tubercle** with the transverse process of the corresponding vertebra. The two articular regions act like a hinge, forcing the rib to move through an axis passing through these areas. The flattened shaft of the rib is weakest at the **angle of the rib** and this is where it tends to fracture in an adult. The upper two ribs, protected by the clavicle and the two floating ribs are least likely to fracture. There is a cervical rib attached to the transverse process of C7 in 0.5% of people and the presence of this rib may cause paraesthesiae or vascular problems, due to pressure on the brachial plexus or subclavian artery.

Intercostal spaces contain **external intercostal muscles** whose fibres pass downwards and forwards between the ribs, **internal intercostal muscles** whose fibres pass downwards and backwards and an incomplete **innermost intercostal layer** (Fig. 2c). They are innervated by **intercostal nerves**, which are the anterior primary rami of **thoracic nerves**. **Intercostal veins, arteries** and **nerves** lie in grooves on the undersurface of the corresponding rib, with the vein above, artery in the middle and nerve below.

The dome-shaped **diaphragm** (Fig. 2d) separates the thorax and abdomen and consists of a muscular peripheral part and a **central tendon**, which is partly fused with the pericardium. The muscular diaphragm takes its origin from the vertebrae and arcuate ligaments, the rib cage and the sternum. The **right crus** arises from the upper three lumbar vertebrae and the **left crus** from the upper two lumbar vertebrae. Their fibrous medial borders form the **median arcuate ligament** over the front of the aorta. The **medial and lateral arcuate ligaments** are thickenings of the fascia overlying the psoas major and quadratus lumborum, respectively. The costal part of the diaphragm is attached to the inner aspects of the 7th to 12th ribs and costal cartilages. The sternal part originates as two slips from the back of the xiphisternum. The **phrenic nerves (C3, 4, 5)** supply motor fibres. Sensory innervation of the central diaphragm also runs in the phrenic, and pain from irritation of the diaphragm is often referred to the corresponding dermatome for C4, the shoulder-tip. The lower intercostal nerves supply sensory fibres to the peripheral diaphragm. The aorta, thoracic duct and azygos vein pass through the diaphragm at the aortic opening at the level of T12. The oesophagus, branches of the left gastric artery and vein and both vagi pass through the oesophageal opening at the level of T10, and the inferior vena cava and right phrenic nerve pass through an opening at the level of T8.

Muscles of respiration

Inspiratory muscles all act to increase thoracic volume, causing intrapleural and alveolar pressure to fall to create an alveolar-to-mouth pressure gradient, drawing air into the lungs. The domes of the **diaphragm**, the main inspiratory muscle, move down when it contracts, by about 1.5 cm during quiet breathing and 6–7 cm during deep breathing. During quiet breathing, the first rib remains fairly still and the **external intercostals** elevate and evert the succeeding ribs, increasing both the anterior–posterior and transverse diameters of the chest wall, the so-called 'bucket-handle' action. The expanded chest wall and lungs will recoil by themselves and quiet breathing uses no expiratory muscles.

When ventilation or resistance to breathing is increased, **accessory inspiratory muscles** aid inspiration. These include the **scalene muscles, sternomastoids** and **serratus anterior**. If the arms are fixed by grasping the edge of a table, contraction of the **pectoralis major**, which normally adducts the arm, helps expand the chest. When ventilation exceeds about 40 L/min, there is activation of expiratory muscles, especially **abdominal muscles (rectus abdominis, external and internal oblique)**, which speed up recoil of the diaphragm by raising intra-abdominal pressure.

In quiet breathing ventilation is largely diaphragmatic, but when the phrenic nerves are damaged, normal ventilation can be maintained by the intercostal muscles. In a high cervical cord transection all respiratory muscles are paralysed, but when the damage is below the phrenic nerve roots (C3, 4, 5) breathing continues via the diaphragm alone. In the newborn, ribs are horizontal, so rib movements cannot increase the volume of the chest and breathing is entirely by the up-and-down action of the diaphragm or so-called **abdominal breathing**. As the ribs become more oblique with increasing age, the movement of the ribs becomes more important to give **thoracic breathing**.

3 Pressures and volumes during normal breathing

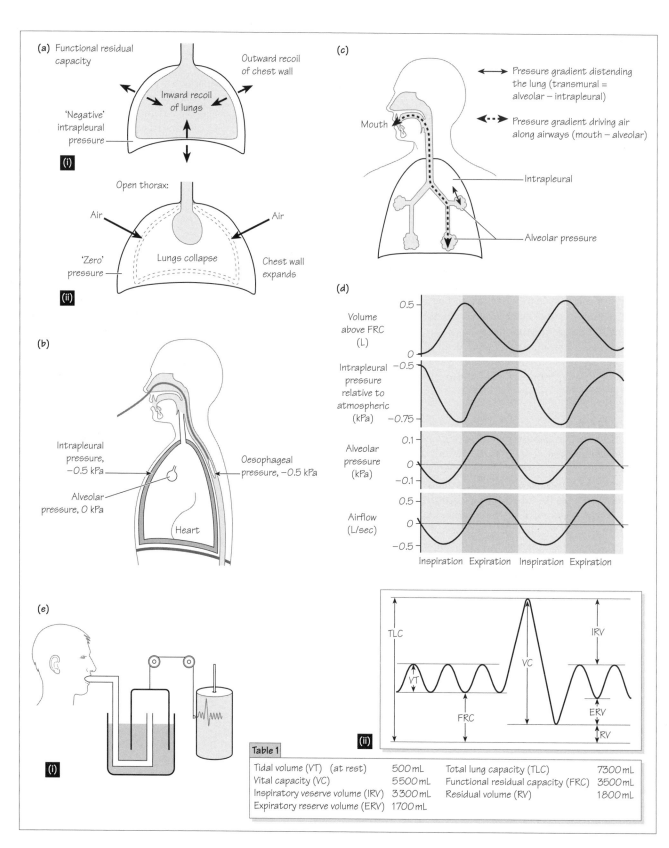

(a) Functional residual capacity

Outward recoil of chest wall

Inward recoil of lungs

'Negative' intrapleural pressure

(i)

Open thorax:

Air

Air

'Zero' pressure

Lungs collapse

Chest wall expands

(ii)

(b)

Intrapleural pressure, −0.5 kPa

Oesophageal pressure, −0.5 kPa

Alveolar pressure, 0 kPa

Heart

(c)

Mouth

Pressure gradient distending the lung (transmural = alveolar − intrapleural)

Pressure gradient driving air along airways (mouth − alveolar)

Intrapleural

Alveolar pressure

(d)

Volume above FRC (L)   0.5   0

Intrapleural pressure relative to atmospheric (kPa)   −0.5   −0.75

Alveolar pressure (kPa)   0.1   0   −0.1

Airflow (L/sec)   0.5   0   −0.5

Inspiration Expiration Inspiration Expiration

(e)

(i)

(ii)

TLC   IRV

VC

VT

FRC   ERV

RV

Table 1

Tidal volume (VT) (at rest)	500 mL	Total lung capacity (TLC)	7300 mL
Vital capacity (VC)	5500 mL	Functional residual capacity (FRC)	3500 mL
Inspiratory veserve volume (IRV)	3300 mL	Residual volume (RV)	1800 mL
Expiratory reserve volume (ERV)	1700 mL		

Functional residual capacity

The volume left in the lungs at the end of a normal breath is known as the **functional residual capacity (FRC)**. At FRC, the respiratory muscles are relaxed and its volume is determined by the elastic properties of the lungs and chest wall.

The lungs are elastic bodies whose resting volume when removed from the body is very small. The natural resting position of the chest wall, seen when the chest is opened surgically, is about 1 L larger than at the end of a normal breath.

In the living respiratory system, the lungs are sealed within the chest wall. Between these two elastic structures is the **intrapleural space**, which contains only a few millilitres of fluid. When the respiratory muscles are relaxed the lungs and chest wall recoil in opposite directions, creating a subatmospheric ('negative') pressure in the space between them, and this tends to oppose the recoil of both the lungs and chest wall. **Functional residual capacity** occurs when the **outward recoil** of the chest wall exactly balances the **inward recoil** of the lungs (Fig. 3a). When the chest is opened, air enters the intrapleural space, the pressure becomes atmospheric and nothing opposes the recoil of the lungs and chest wall. The lungs shrink to a small volume and the chest wall springs out.

If the elastic recoil of either the lungs or chest wall is abnormally large or small, FRC will be abnormal. In lung fibrosis, the lungs are stiff and have increased elastic recoil, so the balance point, and hence FRC, occurs at a small lung volume. In emphysema, there is loss of alveolar tissue and with it, loss of elastic recoil. When the respiratory muscles are relaxed, the reduced elastic recoil of the lungs offers less opposition to the outward recoil of the chest wall and FRC is increased (**barrel chest**). Increased FRC can also occur because of 'air trapping' (see Chapter 7).

Intrapleural pressure

The space between the **visceral pleura** lining the lungs and the **parietal pleura** lining the chest wall is so small that measuring **intrapleural pressure** with a needle risks puncturing the lung. Intrapleural pressure can be indirectly assessed from **oesophageal pressure** (Fig. 3b). The oesophagus is normally closed at the top and bottom except during swallowing and in the upright subject the oesophageal pressure is the same as in the neighbouring intrapleural space. The subject swallows a balloon containing a little air and its pressure is measured via a tube connected to a manometer. Gravity affects the fluid-lined intrapleural space and at FRC in an upright subject, the intrapleural pressure at the apex of the lungs is about $-0.5\,kPa$ ($-5\,cm\,H_2O$) and about $-0.2\,kPa$ ($-2\,cm\,H_2O$) at the bottom.

Pressures, flow and volume during a normal breathing cycle

During inspiration, the chest wall is expanded and intrapleural pressure falls. This increases the pressure gradient between the intrapleural space and alveoli (Fig. 3c), stretching the lungs. The alveoli expand and **alveolar pressure** falls, creating a pressure gradient between the mouth and alveoli, causing air to flow into the lungs. The airflow profile (Fig. 3d) closely follows that of alveolar pressure. During expiration, both intrapleural pressure and alveolar pressure rise. In quiet breathing, intrapleural pressure remains negative for the whole respiratory cycle, whereas alveolar pressure is negative during inspiration and positive during expiration. Alveolar pressure is always higher than intrapleural, because of the recoil of the lung. It is zero at the end of both inspiration and expiration and airflow ceases momentarily. When ventilation is increased, the changes of intrapleural and alveolar pressure are greater and in expiration intrapleural pressure may rise above atmospheric. In forced expiration, coughing or sneezing, intrapleural pressure may rise to $+8\,kPa$ or more.

Lung volumes

If a subject breathes in and out of a **simple water-filled spirometer** (Fig. 3e (i)), the drum falls and rises and the pen, attached by a pulley system, produces a trace (Fig. 3e (ii)). The volume breathed in (or out) is known as the **tidal volume** and the trace shows several **resting tidal volumes,** which are typically about 500 mL. For the fourth breath, the subject breathes in and out as fully as possible. This maximum tidal volume is the **vital capacity**. At the end of a normal quiet inspiration, the subject could breathe in more and this is the **inspiratory reserve volume**. Similarly, the volume that he or she could exhale after a normal expiration is the **expiratory reserve volume**. At the end of a maximal breath out, the volume remaining is the **residual volume. Functional residual capacity** and **total lung capacity** are the volumes in the lungs at the end of a normal expiration and after a maximal breath in, respectively. Typical values in an adult male are given in Table 1. Although a zero volume line is shown (Fig. 3e (ii)), it is not possible to know where this actually is on a trace, because the subject cannot empty the lungs into the drum. For this reason, although illustrated in Fig. 3e (ii), volumes on the right of Table 1 cannot be measured from a simple spirometer trace. They can be measured using **helium dilution** or **body plethysmography** (Chapter 18). The range of normal lung volumes is large and an individual's volumes must be assessed with the aid of **nomograms** that give the predicted value of each volume for the subject's age, sex and height.

4 Gas laws and respiratory symbols

(a) Standard respiratory symbols

Primary symbols

F = Fractional concentration of gas   P = Pressure or partial pressure
C = Content of a gas in blood   S = Saturation of haemoglobin with oxygen
V = Volume of a gas   Q = Volume of blood

A dot over a letter means a time derivative, e.g. $\dot{V}$ = Ventilation (L/min)
$\qquad\qquad\qquad\qquad\qquad\qquad\qquad\qquad\quad \dot{Q}$ = Blood flow (L/min)

Secondary symbols

Gas: I = Inspired gas   **Blood:** a = Arterial
$\qquad$ E = Expired gas $\qquad\quad$ v = Venous
$\qquad$ A = Alveolar gas $\qquad\quad$ c = Capillary
$\qquad$ D = Dead space gas $\qquad\quad$ A dash means mixed or mean
$\qquad$ T = Tidal $\qquad\qquad\quad$ e.g. $\bar{v}$ = Mixed venous
$\qquad$ B = Barometric $\qquad\quad$ A ' after a symbol means end
$\qquad$ ET = End-tidal $\qquad\qquad\quad$ e.g. c' = End-capillary

Tertiary symbols   Examples

O_2 = Oxygen $\dot{V}O_2$ = Oxygen consumption
CO_2 = Carbon dioxide P_{ACO_2} = Alveolar partial pressure
CO = Carbon monoxide $\qquad\qquad$ of carbon dioxide

(b) Correction factors for gas volumes

$$\text{Volume}_{(BTPS)} = \text{volume}_{(ATPS)} \left(\frac{273 + 37}{273 + t^0C}\right)\left(\frac{P_B - P_{H_2O}}{P_B - 6.3*}\right) \quad *47 \text{ if } P_B \text{ and } P_{H_2O} \text{ are in mmHg}$$

$$\text{Volume}_{(STPD)} = \text{volume}_{(ATPS)} \left(\frac{273}{273 + t^0C}\right)\left(\frac{P_B - P_{H_2O}}{101*}\right) \quad *760 \text{ if } P_B \text{ and } P_{H_2O} \text{ are in mmHg}$$

(c) Partial pressure of a gas in a liquid

Gas
phase, Pg

Liquid
phase
liquid X,
PXg

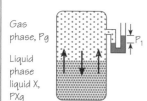 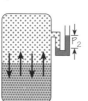 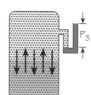

Gas
phase, Pg

Liquid
phase
liquid Y,
PYg

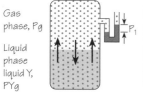 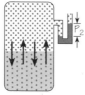 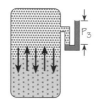

Liquid X containing dissolved gas, g, is exposed to a gas phase containing g at three different partial pressures, P_1, P_2, P_3. Only when the Pg = P_2 does the number of gas molecules leaving the liquid per minute (↑) equal the number entering the liquid (↓) – i.e. the liquid and gas phases are in equilibrium.

∴ Partial pressure of gas, g, in liquid X (PXg) = P_2

Liquid Y also contains gas, g and is also in equilibrium with the gas phase when Pg = P_2

∴ Partial pressure of gas, g, in liquid Y (PYg) = P_2

However, the solubility of gas, g, in liquid Y is less than in liquid X, so at the same partial pressure, liquid Y contains a lower concentration of g.

Note: In the bottom left flask, gas moves against its concentration gradient.

To understand the processes involved in respiration and how valid measurements are made, it is important to understand the behaviour of gases in both gas mixtures and in liquids.

Fractional concentration and partial pressure of gases in the gas mixture

Dalton's law states that when two or more gases, which do not react chemically, are present in the same container, the total pressure is the sum of the partial pressures (the pressure that each gas would exert if isolated in the container).

The total pressure exerted by the atmosphere was traditionally measured by inverting a long mercury-filled glass tube over a mercury reservoir. At sea level, the height of the column supported is normally about 760 mmHg (torr), which in SI units is about 101 kPa (1 kPa = 7.50 mmHg). Dried air contains 21% oxygen. The remaining gases are nitrogen, 78.1%, and inert gases such as argon and helium, 0.9%, although for convenience these physiologically inert gases are often pooled as 'nitrogen, 79%'. Air is considered to be CO_2-free, as the amount present (0.04%) is very small. Standardized symbols used in respiratory physiology are shown in Fig. 4a.

According to Dalton's law:

Dry partial pressure oxygen in inspired air (PIO_2)
= oxygen fraction (FO_2) × total barometric pressure (PB)
= 0.21 × 101 (760) = 21.2 kPa (159 mmHg)

At **altitude**, the oxygen fraction of air is unaltered but barometric pressure is reduced, being about 33.6 kPa (252 mmHg) on the top of Everest.

Water vapour pressure

Air contains variable amounts of water vapour, depending on the water it has been exposed to and the temperature. The maximum or **saturated water vapour pressure** is higher in warm than cool air: at 20°C, it is 2.33 kPa (17.5 mmHg), whereas at body temperature (37°C), it is 6.3 kPa (47 mmHg). The **relative humidity** (actual/saturated water vapour pressure × 100%) of inspired air varies with climate; if it is 40% at 20°C, water vapour pressure will be 0.9 kPa (7 mmHg). The presence of water vapour means that ambient FO_2 and FN_2 are usually a little lower than the dry fractions given above. Air passing down the airways quickly reaches body temperature (37°C) and 100% saturation. Total pressure remains close to barometric, so the added water vapour causes significant dilution of the other gases. The available pressure for the other gases is therefore PB −6.3 kPa (PB −47 mmHg).

The **partial pressure of moist inspired oxygen** (PIO_2) = 0.21 × (PB − saturated vapour pressure at 37°C). At sea level, this is 19.9 kPa (= 0.21 × (101 − 6.3)) or 149.7 mmHg. At altitude, as PB falls, the dilution of inspired gas with water vapour becomes relatively more important. On the top of Everest, where PB is about 33.6 kPa (252 mmHg), moist PIO_2 is 5.7 kPa (43 mmHg).

The effect of pressure and temperature on gas volumes

The inverse relationship between the volume of a perfect gas and its pressure, described by **Boyle's law** ($P \propto 1/V$) and the direct relationship between volume and absolute temperature ($= 273 + °C$) described by **Charles' law ($V \propto T$)** are important when measuring gas volumes. Gas collected in a bag or spirometer will shrink, both because of the direct effect of falling temperature (Charles' law) and because water vapour condenses as temperature falls. To enable valid comparisons, volumes at **ambient temperature and pressure saturated with water (ATPS)** are corrected to those they would occupy under standard conditions. For measurements of lung volumes, this is to **body temperature and pressure saturated with water (BTPS)**. For O_2 consumption or CO_2 production, **standard temperature and pressure dry (STPD)** (0°C, 101.3 kPa (760 mmHg), $PH_2O = 0$) are usually used, so that each litre contains the same number of molecules (1 mole ≈ 22.4 L).

Boyle's law, Charles' law and the reduction of saturated vapour pressure with temperature are combined in the equations for correcting volumes given in Fig. 4b.

Gases dissolved in liquids

If a gas is exposed to a liquid to which it does not react, gas particles will move into the liquid. **Henry's law** states that the number of molecules dissolving in the liquid is directly proportional to the partial pressure at the surface of the gas.

The constant of proportionality is the solubility of the gas in the liquid and it is affected by the gas, the liquid and the temperature, tending to fall as temperature rises.

Content of dissolved gas X in a liquid Y
= solubility of X in Y × partial pressure of X at surface

The **partial pressure of a gas in a liquid** or **gas tension**, is a more difficult concept than that of partial pressure in a gas phase, where we can visualize the pressure of the molecules holding up a column of mercury. The molecules of the gas in the liquid phase will move about in the liquid and have a tendency to escape from the surface, which can be opposed by molecules of the same gas in a gas phase in contact with the liquid (Fig. 4c). If the partial pressure of the gas in the gas phase is altered until there is no net movement of gas between the gas phase and the liquid phase, the gas and liquid are said to be in equilibrium. By definition, the partial pressure of a gas in a liquid is equal to the partial pressure of that gas in a gas phase with which it is in equilibrium. Partial pressure gradient (not concentration gradient) always determines the direction of movement between phases such as a gas and liquid phase.

Note on time derivative symbols

Time derivatives are properly denoted by a dot over the symbol (e.g. $\dot{V}A$, alveolar ventilation in L/min, See Fig. 4a). However, for terms such as the ventilation/perfusion ratio (VA/Q) the dots are often omitted, and this convention is followed throughout this book.

5 Diffusion

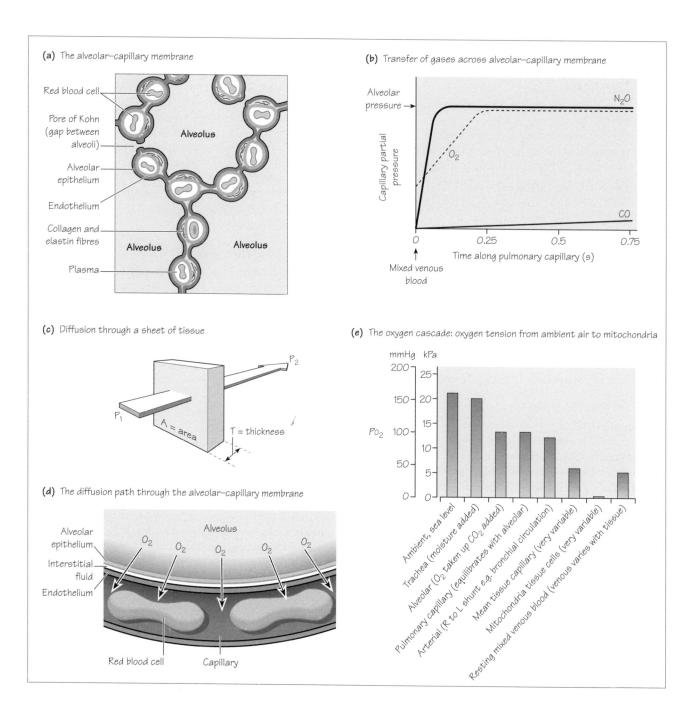

(a) The alveolar–capillary membrane

Red blood cell

Pore of Kohn (gap between alveoli)

Alveolus

Alveolar epithelium

Endothelium

Collagen and elastin fibres

Alveolus

Alveolus

Plasma

(b) Transfer of gases across alveolar–capillary membrane

Alveolar pressure

Capillary partial pressure

N_2O

O_2

CO

Time along pulmonary capillary (s)

Mixed venous blood

(c) Diffusion through a sheet of tissue

P_2

P_1

A = area

T = thickness

(d) The diffusion path through the alveolar–capillary membrane

Alveolar epithelium

Interstitial fluid

Endothelium

Alveolus

O_2 O_2 O_2 O_2 O_2

Red blood cell

Capillary

(e) The oxygen cascade: oxygen tension from ambient air to mitochondria

mmHg kPa

P_{O_2}

Ambient, sea level

Trachea (moisture added)

Alveolar (O_2 taken up CO_2 added)

Pulmonary capillary (equilibrates with alveolar)

Arterial (R to L shunt e.g. bronchial circulation)

Mean tissue capillary (very variable)

Mitochondria tissue cells (very variable)

Resting mixed venous blood (venous varies with tissue)

Oxygen and carbon dioxide are transported in the body by a mixture of **bulk flow** and **diffusion**. Bulk flow, generated by differences in total fluid pressure, is important in most of the airways and in transporting blood containing these gases between pulmonary and tissue capillaries. Diffusion, driven by partial pressure differences, is important in the last few millimetres of the airways, across the alveolar–capillary membrane and between tissue capillaries and mitochondria.

The alveolar–capillary membrane (Fig. 5a)

There are about 300 million alveoli, approximately 0.2 mm in diameter, in an adult male. The wall between alveoli consists of two layers of **alveolar epithelium** resting on two separate basement membranes enclosing the interstitial space, containing **pulmonary capillaries**, elastin and **collagen fibres**. Together, the **alveolar epithelium** and **capillary endothelium** form the **alveolar–capillary membrane**, through which gases diffuse. The alveolar–capillary

18

membrane is very thin (<0.4 μm), except where collagen and elastin fibres are concentrated, with a total surface area of about 85 m^2. The alveolar epithelium has two main types of cell. Type I cells line the alveoli and are relatively devoid of organelles. Type II alveolar cells are rounded with large nuclei, microvilli and cytoplasm containing striated osmiophilic lamellar bodies which store surfactant, an important component of alveolar lining fluid (Chapter 6).

Diffusion and perfusion limitation (Fig. 5b)

If gas containing the poorly soluble gas nitrous oxide (N_2O) is inhaled, pulmonary capillary PN_2O rises and quickly equilibrates with alveolar PN_2O. With no alveolar–capillary partial pressure gradient remaining, diffusion ceases for the rest of the pulmonary capillary and uptake can only be increased by increasing pulmonary capillary blood flow. N_2O uptake is said to be **perfusion-limited**. In contrast, when a mixture containing carbon monoxide (CO) is breathed, the CO combines so avidly with haemoglobin that pulmonary capillary PCO rises little. The pressure gradient driving diffusion is preserved along the capillary. CO uptake would not be increased by increased perfusion, but it would be if diffusion resistance was reduced by reduced thickness or increased area of the alveolar–capillary membrane. CO transfer is **diffusion-limited**. Oxygen transfer lies between these two extremes, but is normally perfusion-limited.

Factors affecting diffusion across a membrane (Fick and Graham's laws)

For a sheet of tissue of area A and thickness T through which gas G is passing (Fig. 5c):

$$\text{Rate of transfer of gas G} \propto \frac{A}{T}(P_1 - P_2)$$

The constant of proportionality

$$= \frac{\text{solubility of the gas in the membrane(s)}}{\sqrt{\text{Molecular weight of the gas (mw)}}}$$

Although the molecular weight of CO_2 is about 1.4 times that of O_2, it is about 20 times more soluble, and so diffuses more easily.

For the alveolar–capillary membrane, the pressure gradient driving diffusion is alveolar (P_A) minus mean pulmonary capillary ($P_{\bar{c}}$). The constants (s, mw, A and T) can be combined to give a single constant, the **diffusing capacity (D_Lg)** of the lungs for gas, g:

$$\text{Rate of transfer of gas, g} = D_L g(P_A - P\bar{c})$$

Oxygen diffusing capacity, $D_L O_2$

$$= \frac{\text{Oxygen uptake from the lungs } (\dot{V}O_2)}{P_A O_2 - P_{\bar{c}} O_2}$$

Oxygen uptake per unit partial pressure gradient ($D_L O_2$) is affected by the rate of combination with haemoglobin as well as by resistance to diffusion, and so some prefer to call this constant the transfer factor ($T_L O_2$).

Although measurement of $D_L O_2$ is desirable, it is not possible because mean capillary PO_2 ($P_{\bar{c}} O_2$) cannot be measured.

Carbon monoxide diffusing capacity, $D_L CO$

$$= \frac{\text{CO uptake from the lungs } (\dot{V}CO)}{P_A CO - P_{\bar{c}} CO}$$

CO diffuses through the same pathway as O_2 and its rate of diffusion is affected by the same factors that affect oxygen transfer. However, unlike $D_L O_2$, $D_L CO$ is measurable. Once CO arrives in the pulmonary capillary blood, it too combines with haemoglobin. Haemoglobin has approximately 240 times the affinity for CO than it does for O_2 and consequently as CO is transferred, almost all of it enters chemical combination and the mean pulmonary capillary PCO can be assumed to be zero.

This simplifies the equation to:

$$D_L CO = \frac{\text{Carbon monoxide uptake from the lungs } (\dot{V}CO)}{P_A CO}$$

Several methods are used for measuring $D_L CO$, but all involve breathing a low level of CO (e.g. 0.3%). Helium is included as a measure of dilution by alveolar gas. By sampling exhaled gas, CO uptake and mean alveolar PCO can be calculated. The normal value depends on the method used, but is about 15–30 mL/min/mmHg (112–225 mL/min/kPa). $D_L CO$ is sometimes divided by alveolar volume to give an index ($K CO$) that corrects for different lung volumes.

Factors affecting $D_L CO$

$D_L CO$ is reduced by a reduction in alveolar–capillary membrane area in emphysema, pulmonary emboli or lung resection and by increased thickness in pulmonary oedema. In pulmonary fibrosis, diffusion is impaired both by thickening of the alveolar–capillary membrane and by the reduced area caused by reduced lung volume. Increased pulmonary blood volume, as occurs in exercise, increases the effective area and $D_L CO$. $D_L CO$ is increased with polycythaemia and reduced in anaemia. $D_L CO$ is therefore non-specific and not diagnostic of any particular condition. Its value lies in its sensitivity to abnormality, which it may reveal when other lung function tests are normal. In hypoventilation, reduced $P_A CO$ causes reduced CO uptake and $D_L CO$ is unaffected.

The oxygen cascade (Fig. 5e) shows how PO_2 falls between air and mitochondria. Mitochondrial oxidative phosphorylation will cease when PO_2 falls below 1 mmHg (0.13 kPa) and this ultimately limits the capillary PO_2 that can be tolerated and therefore the amount of oxygen that can be removed as blood passes through the tissues. Capillary PO_2 must remain high enough to drive diffusion to cells at a rate sufficient to match oxygen consumption and maintain mitochondrial PO_2 above this critical level.

6 Lung mechanics: elastic forces

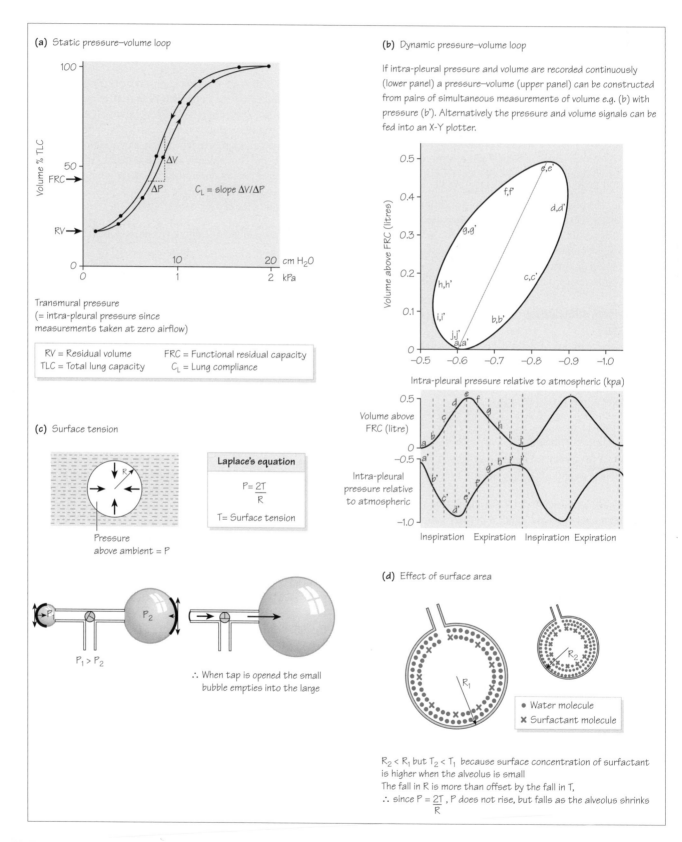

(a) Static pressure–volume loop

Volume % TLC

C_L = slope $\Delta V/\Delta P$

Transmural pressure
(= intra-pleural pressure since
measurements taken at zero airflow)

| RV = Residual volume | FRC = Functional residual capacity |
| TLC = Total lung capacity | C_L = Lung compliance |

(b) Dynamic pressure–volume loop

If intra-pleural pressure and volume are recorded continuously
(lower panel) a pressure–volume (upper panel) can be constructed
from pairs of simultaneous measurements of volume e.g. (b) with
pressure (b'). Alternatively the pressure and volume signals can be
fed into an X-Y plotter.

Volume above FRC (litres)

Intra-pleural pressure relative to atmospheric (kpa)

Volume above
FRC (litre)

Intra-pleural
pressure relative
to atmospheric

Inspiration   Expiration   Inspiration   Expiration

(c) Surface tension

Laplace's equation

$$P = \frac{2T}{R}$$

T = Surface tension

Pressure
above ambient = P

$P_1 > P_2$

∴ When tap is opened the small
bubble empties into the large

(d) Effect of surface area

- Water molecule
- ✖ Surfactant molecule

$R_2 < R_1$ but $T_2 < T_1$ because surface concentration of surfactant
is higher when the alveolus is small
The fall in R is more than offset by the fall in T,
∴ since $P = \frac{2T}{R}$, P does not rise, but falls as the alveolus shrinks

To breathe in, the inspiratory muscles must contract to overcome the impedance offered by the lungs and chest wall. This is mainly in the form of frictional **airway resistance** (Chapter 7) and **elastic resistance** to stretching of the lung and chest wall tissues and the fluid lining the alveoli.

Assessing the stiffness of the lungs: lung compliance

The 'stretchiness' of the lung is usually assessed as lung compliance (C_L) which is the change in lung volume per unit change in distending pressure ($C_L = \Delta V/\Delta P$). The distending pressure, P, is the pressure difference across the lung, which equals alveolar − intrapleural pressure.

Intrapleural pressure can be assessed using an oesophageal balloon (Chapter 3). Alveolar pressure cannot easily be measured directly, but when no air is flowing alveolar pressure must equal mouth pressure (i.e. zero). The transmural pressure, P, is then equal to −intrapleural pressure. The subject breathes in steps and measurements are taken while the breath is held and plotted as a **static pressure–volume (P–V) curve** (Fig. 6a). The curve flattens as the lung volume approaches total lung capacity. The inspiratory curve is slightly different from the expiratory curve and this **hysteresis** is a common property of elastic bodies. **Static lung compliance** is the slope of the steepest part of this static pressure–volume curve in the region just above functional residual capacity (FRC).

Lung compliance is normally about 1.5 L/kPa, but as with lung volumes it is affected by the subject's size, age and sex. In **restrictive disease**, such as lung fibrosis, lung compliance is low. Like a stiff spring, once stretched, fibrosed lungs have an increased tendency to shrink back to their resting position or increased **elastic recoil**. The loss of alveolar tissue in **emphysema** makes them easier to stretch and lung compliance is increased. Although safe, swallowing an oesophageal balloon is not very pleasant or convenient. Fortunately, it is often possible to deduce that a patient has stiff lungs from other measurements such as **FRC** (Chapter 3, 17 and 24), forced expiratory volume in 1 s (**FEV$_1$**) and forced vital capacity (**FVC**) (Chapter 17).

Dynamic pressure–volume loops and dynamic compliance

A **dynamic pressure–volume loop** (upper panel of Fig. 6b) is obtained from continuous measurements of intrapleural pressure and volume during a normal breathing cycle (lower panel of Fig. 6b). There are two points, at the ends of inspiration and expiration, where airflow and alveolar pressure are zero (a, a′ and e, e′) and the slope of the line joining these points is **dynamic compliance**. In health, its value is similar to the **static compliance,** but in some diseases it may be lower, as stiff areas may fill preferentially during normal breathing. Between the two zero flow points, the dynamic P–V loop appears fatter than the static P–V loop, as intrapleural pressure must change more to drive airflow. In fact, the area of the dynamic loop is a measure of the work done against airway resistance (Chapter 7).

The air–fluid interface lining the alveoli

During inspiration, as well as stretching the collagen and elastin fibres, the **surface tension** forces at the air–alveolar lining fluid interface must be overcome. At the surface of a bubble, the attraction of the fluid molecules for each other creates a tension, which tends to shrink the bubble (Fig. 6c). LaPlace discovered that a gas bubble in a liquid would shrink until the pressure, P, within it reached a value of 2T/R, where T is a constant, the surface tension of the fluid and R the radius of the bubble. The **law of Laplace (P = 2T/R)** predicts that if two bubbles are made of the same fluid, the smaller bubble will have a higher pressure within it—since when the radius of curvature is small, a greater proportion of the surface tension is directed to the centre of the bubble (lower panel of Fig. 6.1c). When the two bubbles are connected, the small bubble empties into the large bubble as air flows down the pressure gradient.

The presence of an air–fluid interface creates several potential problems:

1 It reduces lung compliance and the higher the surface tension the lower the compliance.

2 The alveoli would be inherently unstable, with the smaller alveoli tending to collapse completely.

3 As the fluid tends to shrink away from the alveolar cells, it would create a suction force tending to cause **transudation** of fluid from the nearby pulmonary capillaries.

The absence of these problems in normal adults is thought to be partly due to the presence in the alveolar lining fluid of **surfactant**.

Surfactant

Pulmonary surfactant is a mixture of **phospholipids** such as **sphingomyelin** and **lecithin** produced by the **type II alveolar cells** (Chapter 5). The presence of these substances in the **alveolar lining fluid** lowers the surface tension and increases compliance. The phospholipids have a **hydrophilic** end that lies in the alveolar fluid and a **hydrophobic** end that projects into the alveolar gas and as a result they float on the surface of the lining fluid. As an alveolus shrinks, its surface area diminishes and the surface concentration of surfactant rises (Fig. 6d). As surface tension falls with increasing surface concentration of surfactant, the increased tendency for alveoli to collapse when they shrink is offset and stability improved. Alveolar stability is also aided by the connection and mutual pull of neighbouring alveoli, a phenomenon known as **alveolar interdependence**.

Surfactant production in the fetus gradually increases in the last third of pregnancy and may be inadequate in babies born prematurely, giving rise to the typical problems of **neonatal respiratory distress syndrome (NRDS)**—stiff lungs, areas of collapse and transudation of fluid (Chapter 16).

7 Lung mechanics: airway resistance

(a) Laminar and turbulent flow

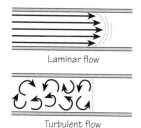

Laminar flow

Turbulent flow

(b) Main factors influencing bronchomotor tone

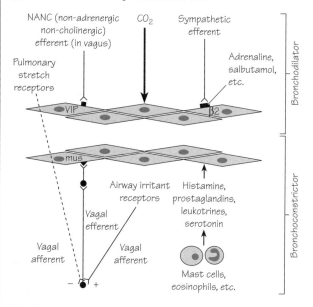

NANC (non-adrenergic non-cholinergic) efferent (in vagus)

CO_2

Sympathetic efferent

Adrenaline, salbutamol, etc.

Pulmonary stretch receptors

VIP

β2

Bronchodilator

mus

Airway irritant receptors

Histamine, prostaglandins, leukotrines, serotonin

Vagal efferent

Vagal afferent

Vagal afferent

Mast cells, eosinophils, etc.

Bronchoconstrictor

β2 = β2 adrenergic receptor, VIP = vasoactive intestinal peptide receptor, mus = muscuranic cholinergic receptor

(d) Dynamic compression of airways

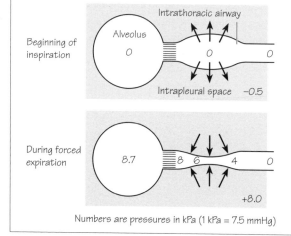

Beginning of inspiration

Alveolus

Intrathoracic airway

0

0

0

Intrapleural space   −0.5

During forced expiration

8.7

8   6   4   0

+8.0

Numbers are pressures in kPa (1 kPa = 7.5 mmHg)

(c) The effect of effort on inspiratory and expiratory airflow

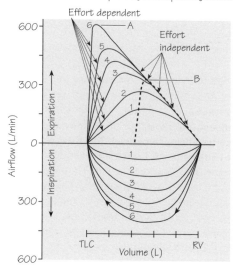

Effort dependent

Effort independent

Airflow (L/min)

Expiration

Inspiration

A

B

TLC

Volume (L)

RV

- - - - = Flow–volume curve for maximum effort from partly filled lungs
A = Peak expiratory flow rate with lungs filled to total lung capacity
B = Peak expiratory flow rate for partly filled lungs filled (RV + 3 litre)
TLC = Total lung capacity, RV = Residual volume

(e) Maximum flow–volume loops

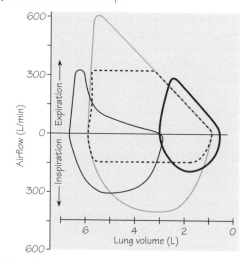

Airflow (L/min)

Expiration

Inspiration

Lung volume (L)

—— **Normal curve**

—— **Obstructive airway disease of smaller airways.** Note:
- concave appearance of forced expiratory curve
- forced inspiratory flow affected less than forced expiratory flow

- - - **Upper airway obstruction (e.g. tracheal stenosis).** Note:
- flat topped flow–volume curve
- forced inspiratory flow affected as much as expiratory flow

—— **Restrictive lung disease.** Low peak flow rates are related to low volume. (Note: this figure is drawn to show the relationship between these traces by using absolute lung volume which cannot actually be obtained from a flow–volume loop alone).

Airflow is driven by the mouth-to-alveolar pressure gradient generated by the respiratory muscles (Chapters 2 and 3).

$$\text{Airflow} = \frac{\Delta P \ (= \text{mouth–alveolar pressure})}{R_{AW} \ (= \text{resistance of the airways})}$$

In **laminar flow**, gas particles move parallel to the walls, with centre layers moving faster than outer ones, creating a cone-shaped front (Fig. 7a). The factors affecting laminar flow of a fluid of viscosity, η, in smooth straight tubes of length, l, and radius, r, are described in **Poiseuille's equation**:

$$\text{Flow} = \frac{\Delta P}{R} = \Delta P \frac{\pi r^4}{8 l \eta} \qquad \therefore R = \frac{8 l \eta}{\pi r^4}$$

Halving the radius of an airway increases its resistance 16-fold. However, although the resistance of an individual bronchiole is high, there are thousands in parallel. The total resistance of each generation of peripheral airways is normally low and the overall resistance of lung airways is dominated by the larger airways. Outside the lung, the nose and pharynx contribute substantial resistance, which can be bypassed by mouth breathing in exercise. Peripheral airways are often affected by disease, but since their resistance must increase considerably to measurably affect airway resistance (RAW) they are known as the **silent zone**.

At higher linear velocities, especially in wide airways and near branch points, flow may become **turbulent**. With turbulence, the wave front is square and flow $\propto \sqrt{\Delta P}$ (not ΔP), reflecting the dissipation of energy in the formation of eddies. Normally, at rest, flow is laminar throughout the airways, but in exercise it may become turbulent, especially in the trachea, generating characteristic harsh breath sounds.

Factors affecting airway resistance
Bronchial smooth muscle and epithelium
Bronchial smooth muscle (Fig. 7b) receives a **parasympathetic bronchoconstrictor** nerve supply, which forms the efferent limb of a reflex from airway irritant receptors. The airways contain β_2-adrenergic receptors, which cause relaxation when stimulated by the sparse sympathetic innervation or more importantly by circulating **epinephrine** (adrenaline) or drugs such as salbutamol. Parasympathetic bronchoconstriction is inhibited by activation of airway stretch receptors and CO_2 has a direct bronchodilator effect. Pollutants (e.g. sulphur dioxide, ozone) and substances released from mast cells and eosinophils can increase RAW via bronchoconstriction, mucosal oedema, mucus hypersecretion, mucus plugging and epithelial shedding, all of which are important in asthma (Chapter 20). Airway resistance can also be increased by chronic mucosal hypertrophy in chronic obstructive pulmonary disease (COPD) (Chapter 22) and by material within the airways, such as inhaled foreign bodies or tumours (Chapter 25).

Transmural (airway — intrapleural) pressure gradient
This can have important effects on airway calibre, and this underlies the effects of effort on airflow illustrated in Fig. 7c. Airflow is measured continuously and plotted against lung volume as the subject breathes between residual volume (RV) and total lung capacity (TLC). The inspiratory airflow at any volume increases progressively with increasing effort (1 = minimum effort, 6 = maximum effort). The flow–volume curves for progressively increasing expiratory efforts (upper traces 1–6) are more complicated. In the early part of expiration from TLC, flow is **effort-dependent**, but towards the end of the breath, as volume declines, the traces produced at different effort levels come together. Expiratory airflow towards the end of a breath is **effort-independent** and determined by lung volume. **Peak expiratory flow rate** (PEFR) is seen to be reduced if the lungs are only partially filled at the start of the forced expiration.

Effort-independent airflow is explained by **dynamic compression of airways**. Before the start of inspiration (Fig. 7d, upper panel) pressure along the airways is zero, intrapleural pressure is negative (Chapter 3), and transmural pressure acts to hold airways open. Intrapleural pressure is negative during both quiet and forced inspiration and it remains negative in quiet expiration, so transmural pressure holds airways open. In a forced expiration, however, expiratory muscle contraction raises intrapleural pressure well above atmospheric (e.g. 8 kPa, 60 mmHg), increasing the pressure gradient from alveoli to mouth. This would be expected to increase airflow, but the increased intrapleural pressure also acts to compress airways. Airway pressure falls progressively along the airway and at some point—usually in the bronchi—the airway pressure will be sufficiently below intrapleural pressure for the airway to collapse, despite its cartilaginous support. Pressure will then build up distally, opening the airways again. The resulting fluttering walls can be seen on bronchoscopy and produce the brassy note audible on forced expiration in normal people.

RAW in disease
Increased airway resistance is important in many diseases and can be measured using a body plethysmograph. In health, RAW is about 0.2 kPa/L/s (1.5 mmHg/L/s). More commonly, airway resistance is assessed indirectly from forced expiratory measurements, such as **forced expiratory volume in 1 s** (FEV_1), **forced vital capacity** (FVC) and PEFR (Chapter 17). High airway resistance accentuates dynamic compression of airways by augmenting the pressure drop along airways. In addition, the airways may be less able to resist compression, in emphysema because of reduced radial traction and in asthma because of bronchoconstriction. Collapse of small airways may occur, leading to incomplete expiration, **air trapping** and increased functional residual capacity. Inability to produce high expiratory airflow impairs effective coughing, which can lead to a vicious cycle as secretions accumulate, further increasing RAW and further reducing peak flow.

Expiratory wheezes (rhonchi), heard in asthma and other obstructive diseases, are probably generated by oscillations in opposing airway walls near their point of closure, like sounds from the reeds of an oboe. A reasonable airflow is needed to generate such sounds and when constriction becomes very severe, they disappear to give the ominous silent chest seen in life-threatening asthma. Small airway collapse leads to characteristic shape of the flow–volume curve in obstructive airway disease (Fig. 7e), which differs from that in upper airway obstruction and restrictive lung disease.

8 Carriage of oxygen

(a) Haemoglobin structure

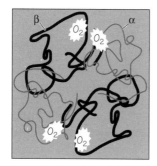

Haemoglobin is composed of four subunits, each containing a protein chain (globin) and a haem group. Normal adult haemoglobin, HbA, contains two identical α-chains composed of 141 amino acids and two β-chains composed of 146 amino acids. The haem group (✿) is attached to each chain at a histidine residue and each has an iron atom in the ferrous form, which binds to an oxygen molecule. The haem groups lie in crevices in the crumpled ball of globin chains. The exact 3D (or quaternary) structure of haemoglobin can change and alter the accessibility of the oxygen binding site. Each molecule of haemoglobin can bind up to four molecules of oxygen in a series of reactions which can be summarized as:

$$Hb_4 + 4O_2 \Leftrightarrow Hb_4(O_2)_4$$

(b) The oxygen – haemoglobin dissociation curve, haemoglobin concentration, 15g/dL

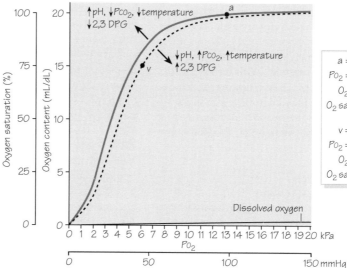

a = Normal arterial blood
Po_2 = 13.3 kPa (100 mmHg)
O_2 content = 20 mL/dL
O_2 saturation = 97%

v = Resting mixed venous
Po_2 = 5.3 kPa (40 mmHg)
O_2 content = 15 mL/dL
O_2 saturation = 75%

(c) Anaemia and carbon monoxide poisoning

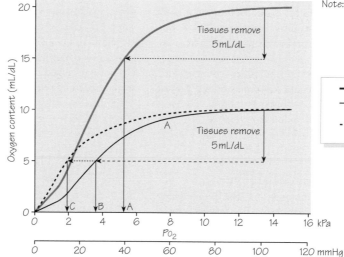

Note: for simplicity the Bohr shift is ignored

Hb = 15 g/dL
Hb = 7.5 g/dL
Hb = 15 g/dL
COHb = 50%

At rest, an adult male consumes about 250 mL oxygen/min, which may rise to more than 4000 mL/min in exercise if he is very fit. Oxygen diffuses from alveolus to blood until equilibrium is reached when pulmonary capillary Po_2 equals alveolar Po_2. The **solubility** of oxygen in blood is low—0.000225 mL oxygen per mL of blood per kPa (0.00003 mL/mL/mmHg)—so that at a normal arterial Po_2 of 13.3 kPa (100 mmHg) there is only 0.3 mL dissolved in each 100 mL of blood. The main function of the red blood cell pigment, **haemoglobin**, whose structure is shown in Fig. 8a, is to carry the large quantities of oxygen needed by the tissues.

Each gram of haemoglobin combines with up to 1.34 mL oxygen, so with a haemoglobin concentration, [Hb], of 15 g/dL, blood contains a maximum of 20 mL/dL oxygen bound to haemoglobin. This is known as the **oxygen capacity**, which varies with [Hb]. The actual amount of oxygen bound also depends on the Po_2. The percentage of the available binding sites bound to oxygen is known as the **oxygen saturation**.

Oxygen saturation

$$= \frac{\text{Amount of oxygen bound to haemoglobin (\textbf{oxygen content}), mL/dL}}{\text{oxygen capacity, mL/dL}} \times 100\%$$

The rate of rise of oxygen content with increasing partial pressure depends on the number of free haemoglobin binding sites remaining and their affinity for oxygen. As each oxygen molecule binds in turn to the four haem groups, the quaternary structure alters and the affinity of the remaining binding sites for oxygen increases. This **cooperative binding** increases the steepness of the **oxygen–haemoglobin dissociation curve** in the middle (Fig. 8b), but the curve flattens again at partial pressures above about 8 kPa (60 mmHg) because there are few remaining sites.

In arterial blood, Po_2 is normally about 13 kPa (100 mmHg) and oxygen saturation about 97%, and with a normal [Hb], an oxygen content about 20 mL/dL. Rises or modest falls in Po_2 from 13 kPa (100 mmHg), for example during hyperventilation or mild hypoventilation, cause little change in the arterial oxygen content, as the dissociation curve is flat in this region. More severe reductions in Po_2, to levels in the steep region, are associated with significant reductions in oxygen saturation and content. Consequently, breathing oxygen-enriched air may significantly raise arterial oxygen content and hence exercise capacity at altitude and in patients with chronic hypoxic respiratory disease, but has little effect on a normal person at sea level.

Low Po_2 in tissue capillaries causes oxygen release from haemoglobin, whereas the high Po_2 in pulmonary capillaries causes oxygen binding. The affinity of haemoglobin for oxygen and hence position of the dissociation curve varies with local conditions. A reduced oxygen affinity, shown by a right shift in the curve, is caused by a fall in pH, a rise in Pco_2 (the **Bohr effect**) or increased temperature (Fig. 8b). These changes occur in metabolically active tissues such as exercising muscle and encourage oxygen release. In the lungs, oxygen uptake is aided by the increasing affinity of haemoglobin for oxygen, caused by falling Pco_2 and temperature and increased pH and reflected by a left shift of the curve. The Po_2 at which the haemoglobin is 50% saturated is known as the $\textbf{P}_{50}$. Under normal arterial conditions (pH=7.4, Pco_2=5.3 kPa or 40 mmHg, temp = 37°C) P_{50}=3.5 kPa (26.3 mmHg); right shifts raise the P_{50} and left shifts lower it. A rise in the concentration of **2,3-di(or bi)phosphoglycerate** (2,3-DPG), which is a by-product of glycolysis in red cells, also causes a right shift. A rise in 2,3-DPG occurs in anaemia, causing a modest increase in P_{50}. Blood bank storage causes progressive depletion of 2,3-DPG and an undesirable left shift, but this can be minimized by storing the blood with citrate-phosphate-dextrose.

In **anaemia**, at any given Po_2, the oxygen content is reduced because of the reduced concentration of binding sites. Figure 8c shows the dissociation curve for normal blood and for blood with [Hb]= 7.5 g/dL. Alveolar and arterial Po_2 is normal in anaemia and therefore arterial O_2 content is 10 mL/dL. At rest, the tissues need to remove about 5 mL/dL from the blood passing through them. To achieve this mixed venous content, Po_2 will need to fall to about 5.3 kPa (40 mmHg) (A in Fig. 8c) when [Hb]=15 g/dL and about 3.6 kPa (mmHg) (B) when [Hb]=7.5 g/dL. The reduced venous and hence capillary Po_2 reduces the partial pressure gradient driving diffusion of oxygen to the tissues, which may become inadequate in exercise when oxygen consumption increases.

Figure 8c also shows the dissociation curve for blood that has 50% of oxygen-binding sites occupied by carbon monoxide (CO, dashed line). Arterial oxygen content is 10 mL/dL, but there is also an altered shape and leftward shift of the dissociation curve, because CO binding increases the affinity of the remaining (CO-free) sites for oxygen. This impairs oxygen release in the tissues. Mixed venous Po_2 will now have to fall to 2 kPa (15 mmHg) (point C) to release the 5 mL/dL required and this will greatly reduce the pressure gradient for diffusion. At about 50–60% **carboxyhaemoglobin**, symptoms of impaired cerebral oxygenation (headache, convulsions, coma and death) develop, whereas anaemic patients with the same arterial oxygen content are typically asymptomatic at rest. Haemoglobin has a high affinity for CO (about 240 times that for oxygen), so breathing even low concentrations causes a progressive increase in the cherry-red carboxyhaemoglobin.

9 Carriage of carbon dioxide

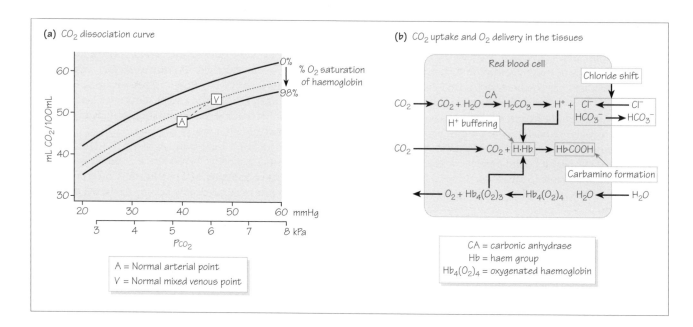

(a) CO_2 dissociation curve

% O_2 saturation of haemoglobin

A = Normal arterial point
V = Normal mixed venous point

(b) CO_2 uptake and O_2 delivery in the tissues

Red blood cell

Chloride shift

H^+ buffering

Carbamino formation

CA = carbonic anhydrase
Hb = haem group
$Hb_4(O_2)_4$ = oxygenated haemoglobin

Carbon dioxide (CO_2) is produced by tissues and transported in the blood to the lungs, where it is expired. The amount of CO_2 that can be carried in the blood is much greater than that of O_2, as seen in the **CO_2 dissociation curve** (Fig. 9a). The CO_2 dissociation curve is also more linear and does not reach a plateau. CO_2 is transported in the blood as bicarbonate ions, as carbamino compounds combined with proteins or simply dissolved in the plasma.

Bicarbonate: About 60% of CO_2 is transported in the form of bicarbonate. CO_2 and water combine to form carbonic acid (H_2CO_3) and thence bicarbonate (HCO_3^-):

$$CO_2 + H_2O \overset{CA}{\Leftrightarrow} H_2CO_3 \Leftrightarrow H^+ + HCO_3^- \qquad (1)$$

The left-hand side of the equation proceeds slowly in plasma, but is accelerated dramatically by the enzyme **carbonic anhydrase** (CA), which is present in red blood cells. Ionization of carbonic acid to bicarbonate and H^+ is rapid in the absence of any enzyme. Bicarbonate is therefore formed preferentially in the red cells, from which it easily diffuses out into the plasma. The red cell membrane is, however, impermeable to H^+ ions and they remain within the cell. In order to maintain electrical neutrality, Cl^- ions diffuse into the cell, an effect known as the **chloride shift** (Fig. 9b). A build-up of H^+ in the red blood cell would impair further movement of equation 1 to the right, thus limiting formation of bicarbonate. However, H^+ binds avidly to reduced (deoxygenated) haemoglobin, i.e. haemoglobin acts as a buffer, so the rise in H^+ concentration is limited and more bicarbonate can be formed. Oxygenated haemoglobin does not bind H^+ so well, as it is more acid. This contributes to the **Haldane effect**, which states that, for any given $P\text{co}_2$, the CO_2 content of deoxygenated blood is greater than that of oxygenated blood. As a result, when blood gives up oxygen to respiring tissues, i.e. becomes deoxygenated, it is able to take up more of the CO_2 that

the tissues are producing. Conversely, oxygenation of haemoglobin in the lung assists the unloading of CO_2 from the blood. This is illustrated by Fig. 9a and equation 2.

$$H^+ + \text{Haemoglobin} \cdot O_2 \Leftrightarrow \text{Haemoglobin} \cdot H + O_2 \qquad (2)$$

Note that as a consequence of all the above, deoxygenated red cells have a higher intracellular osmolality and water enters, causing them to swell slightly. In the lung, CO_2 is given off, osmolality falls and the red cells shrink again.

Carbamino compounds: CO_2 combines rapidly with terminal amino groups on proteins to form carbamino compounds:

$$CO_2 + \text{Protein} \cdot NH_2 \Leftrightarrow \text{Protein} \cdot NH \cdot COOH \qquad (3)$$

In blood, the most prevalent protein is haemoglobin, which combines with CO_2 to form carbaminohaemoglobin. Reduced haemoglobin forms carbamino compounds more readily than oxygenated haemoglobin and this also contributes to the Haldane effect (Fig. 9b). Around 30% of the CO_2 expired by the lungs is carried as carbamino compounds.

CO_2 in solution: CO_2 is ~20 times more soluble in water than O_2. A significant proportion (~10%) of the CO_2 exhaled is therefore carried to the lung dissolved in the plasma.

Hypoventilation and hyperventilation

Ventilation is normally closely matched to the metabolic requirements of the body and this can be estimated from the rate of CO_2 production (Chapter 12). The partial pressure of CO_2 in the alveoli ($P_A\text{co}_2$) is proportional to the amount of CO_2 exhaled per minute ($V\text{co}_2$) as a fraction of total alveolar ventilation (V_A), i.e. $P_A\text{co}_2 \propto V\text{co}_2/V_A$. The gas in the alveoli is in equilibrium with arterial blood, so $P_A\text{CO}_2$ estimates the partial pressure in the blood ($P_a\text{CO}_2$). At any given metabolic rate, doubling the alveolar ventilation halves alveolar and arterial $P\text{CO}_2$, and halving alveolar ventilation doubles $P_A\text{CO}_2$ and $P_a\text{CO}_2$. Changes in alveolar ventilation also affect alveolar $P\text{O}_2$, but the relationship is not as simple because O_2 is present in both inspired and expired gas. Thus doubling alveolar ventilation will halve the *difference* between the inspired and alveolar O_2 fraction. **Hypoventilation** (under-ventilation) and **hyperventilation** (over-ventilation) are therefore defined in terms of $P_a\text{CO}_2$, so that a patient is *hypoventilating* when $P_a\text{CO}_2 > 45$ mmHg (5.9 kPa) and *hyperventilating* when the $P_a\text{CO}_2 < 40$ mmHg (5.3 kPa). Note that the CO_2 content of the blood will be affected more slowly by hypo- or hyperventilation than the O_2 content, as the CO_2 stores in the body (e.g. as HCO_3^-) are ~75 times greater than those for O_2 (e.g. haemoglobin, myoglobin). Also, although hyperventilation increases arterial $P\text{O}_2$, in a healthy patient it has little effect on O_2 content as the haemoglobin is normally close to saturation (Chapter 8).

Hypoventilation may occur when the respiratory drive is impaired by head injury, or drugs such as morphine or barbiturates which suppress the respiratory centres. It may also be caused by respiratory muscle weakness or severe chest trauma. Hypoventilation is sometimes a feature of severe chronic obstructive airways disease (COPD; Chapter 23), but is not usually a feature of asthma (Chapter 21) unless the attack is severe or prolonged enough to lead to exhaustion. Hypoventilation is difficult to achieve voluntarily, as the respiratory centres create an overwhelming desire to breathe. Hyperventilation can be induced voluntarily and in states of high anxiety or pain.

Hypoventilation leads to **hypercapnia** (high $P_a\text{CO}_2$) and **hypoxia** (low $P_a\text{O}_2$). Increasing severity of hypercapnia causes peripheral vasodilatation, muscle twitching and hand flap, confusion, drowsiness and eventually coma; there is a concomitant respiratory acidosis (Chapter 10). The effects of hypoxia are dealt with elsewhere (Chapter 8). A low $P_a\text{CO}_2$ as a result of hyperventilation causes light-headedness, visual disturbances due to cerebral vasoconstriction, paraesthesia ('pins and needles') and muscle cramps, especially carpopedal spasm.

Respiratory gas exchange ratio

Respiratory gas exchange ratio (R) is the ratio of CO_2 production to O_2 consumption as measured at the mouth. In the steady state CO_2 production and O_2 consumption reflect tissue metabolism. Metabolizing carbohydrates produces a volume of CO_2 equal to the volume of O_2 consumed, whereas metabolizing fats and proteins produces a smaller volume of CO_2 than O_2 consumed. For an average mixed diet $R \approx 0.8$.

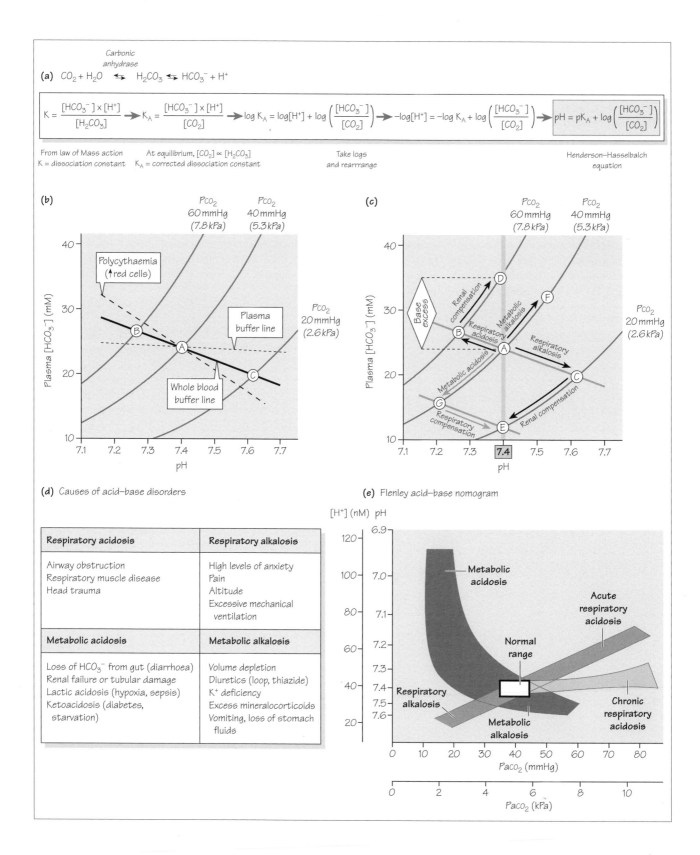

(a)

Carbonic anhydrase

$$CO_2 + H_2O \leftrightarrows H_2CO_3 \leftrightarrows HCO_3^- + H^+$$

$$K = \frac{[HCO_3^-] \times [H^+]}{[H_2CO_3]} \rightarrow K_A = \frac{[HCO_3^-] \times [H^+]}{[CO_2]} \rightarrow \log K_A = \log[H^+] + \log\left(\frac{[HCO_3^-]}{[CO_2]}\right) \rightarrow -\log[H^+] = -\log K_A + \log\left(\frac{[HCO_3^-]}{[CO_2]}\right) \rightarrow pH = pK_A + \log\left(\frac{[HCO_3^-]}{[CO_2]}\right)$$

From law of Mass action   At equilibrium, $[CO_2] \propto [H_2CO_3]$ Take logs   Henderson–Hasselbalch
K = dissociation constant K_A = corrected dissociation constant   and rearrrange   equation

(b)

Pco_2 60 mmHg (7.8 kPa) Pco_2 40 mmHg (5.3 kPa)

Polycythaemia (↑red cells)

Plasma buffer line

Pco_2 20 mmHg (2.6 kPa)

Whole blood buffer line

Plasma $[HCO_3^-]$ (mM)

pH

(c)

Pco_2 60 mmHg (7.8 kPa) Pco_2 40 mmHg (5.3 kPa)

Base excess

Renal compensation

Metabolic alkalosis

Respiratory acidosis

Metabolic acidosis

Respiratory alkalosis

Pco_2 20 mmHg (2.6 kPa)

Respiratory compensation

Renal compensation

Plasma $[HCO_3^-]$ (mM)

7.4

pH

(d) Causes of acid–base disorders

Respiratory acidosis	Respiratory alkalosis
Airway obstruction Respiratory muscle disease Head trauma	High levels of anxiety Pain Altitude Excessive mechanical ventilation
Metabolic acidosis	**Metabolic alkalosis**

Loss of HCO_3^- from gut (diarrhoea)
Renal failure or tubular damage
Lactic acidosis (hypoxia, sepsis)
Ketoacidosis (diabetes,
  starvation)
	Volume depletion
	Diuretics (loop, thiazide)
	K^+ deficiency
	Excess mineralocorticoids
	Vomiting, loss of stomach
	  fluids

(e) Flenley acid–base nomogram

$[H^+]$ (nM) pH

Metabolic acidosis

Acute respiratory acidosis

Normal range

Respiratory alkalosis

Chronic respiratory acidosis

Metabolic alkalosis

$Paco_2$ (mmHg)

$Paco_2$ (kPa)

The pH of arterial blood is normally ~7.4 ($[H^+] = 40\,nM$). Regulation of **acid–base status** so that blood pH remains between 7.35 and 7.45 (45–35 nM) is vital for the correct functioning of the body. Carriage of CO_2 in blood and its removal in the lungs (Chapter 9) has an important influence on acid–base status, as around 100 times more acid equivalents are expired per day in the form of CO_2/carbonic acid than are excreted as fixed acids by the kidneys.

Buffers bind or release H^+ according to the pH; this limits the change in pH that occurs when acid is added. The relationship between the amount of acid equivalent added to a solution containing a buffer and the resultant change in pH is known as the **buffer curve**. Buffers are most effective when pH is close to their pK_A (log of dissociation constant, K_A; see Fig. 10a). The most important buffers in blood are **haemoglobin** and **bicarbonate** (HCO_3^-). CO_2 combines with water to form carbonic acid (H_2CO_3), which dissociates to HCO_3^- and H^+ (Chapter 9). The relationship between pH, P_{CO_2} and $[HCO_3^-]$ is described by the **Henderson–Hasselbalch equation** (Fig. 10a):

$$pH = pK_A + \log\left(\frac{[HCO_3^-]}{[CO_2]}\right)$$

pK_A is 6.1 and $[CO_2]$ can be calculated as $P_{CO_2} \times CO_2$ solubility, which is $0.03\,mmol \cdot L \cdot mmHg^{-1}$ ($0.23\,mmol \cdot L \cdot kPa^{-1}$). In normal blood, $[HCO_3^-]$ is 24 mM and P_{CO_2} 40 mmHg (5.3 kPa) and pH calculates as 7.4. Whatever their actual values, if the ratio $[HCO_3^-]$:$[CO_2]$ remains constant at 20, then pH will remain at 7.4. Although the pK_A of the bicarbonate system (6.1) is further away from blood pH (7.4) than would seem ideal for a buffer, the fact that P_{CO_2} and HCO_3^- can be independently controlled by ventilation (Chapter 9) and the kidneys, respectively, means that in practice it makes an effective buffer system.

Haemoglobin is an important buffer, particularly when deoxygenated (Chapter 9) and significantly improves the buffering capacity of whole blood compared with plasma (Fig. 10b; the steeper the line, the better the buffering). All other **blood proteins** combined have <20% of the buffering capacity of haemoglobin.

Acidosis, alkalosis and compensation

The relationship between pH, HCO_3^- and P_{CO_2} can be portrayed using a **Davenport diagram** (Fig. 10b). HCO_3^- is plotted against pH for given values of P_{CO_2}. The line marked BAC is the **buffer line** for whole blood; in the absence of other changes (e.g. anaemia, polycythaemia), changes in P_{CO_2} alter HCO_3^- and pH along this line. Point A represents normal conditions (pH 7.4, HCO_3^- 24 mM, P_{CO_2} 40 mmHg/5.3 kPa). An acute rise in P_{CO_2} (hypercapnia) due to

hypoventilation (e.g. **acute respiratory failure**) will decrease the $[HCO_3^-]$:P_{CO_2} ratio and consequently pH (see above). This **respiratory acidosis** is represented by a move from A to B (Fig. 10c); A to C represents a **respiratory alkalosis** (e.g. hyperventilation). A sustained respiratory acidosis caused by **chronic respiratory failure** (Chapter 20) can be partially **compensated** by excretion of H^+ (as phosphate and ammonium) and reabsorption of HCO_3^- in the kidneys. The $[HCO_3^-]$:P_{CO_2} ratio is thus largely restored and pH returns towards normal. This **renal compensation** is described by the arrow between B and D (Fig. 10c). Conversely, a respiratory alkalosis may be compensated by increased renal excretion of HCO_3^- (C to E).

The term **metabolic acidosis** (or **alkalosis**) is used when acid–base status is disturbed by changes in HCO_3^- rather than CO_2—as a result, for example, of renal disease or increased H^+ production (Fig. 10d). A **metabolic acidosis** (G) may be partially compensated by increased ventilation and a reduction in P_{CO_2} (G to E), initiated by detection of acid pH by the chemoreceptors (Chapter 12). There can be little **respiratory compensation** for **metabolic alkalosis** (F), as this may require unsustainable falls in ventilation.

Base excess

Measurement of pH alone gives little indication of acid–base status (Fig. 10d); although pH may be normal, P_{CO_2} and $[HCO_3^-]$ may not be (D, E). Measurements of blood pH, P_{CO_2} and P_{O_2} are always taken clinically. **Base excess** or **base deficit** (negative base excess) is the millimole per litre of acid or alkali needed to titrate the blood back to a pH of 7.4. It is normally $0 \pm 2\,mmol/L$. In a pure metabolic acidosis, it is greater than the difference between the actual and normal HCO_3^-, as haemoglobin and buffers must also be titrated. Base excess is normally calculated from the pH and P_{CO_2} automatically by clinical blood gas analysers, corrected for haemoglobin. The example in Fig. 10c is for a fully compensated respiratory acidosis (D) and gives an indication of the degree of renal compensation (i.e. after titration back to pH 7.4). Base excess may be useful for diagnosis, but should be used with caution as a basis for treatment, as the whole-body buffer line may differ significantly from that of blood *in vitro*, due to contributions from interstitial fluids (Fig. 10b).

Metabolic and respiratory acid–base disorders may often be combined, making diagnosis difficult. A common example is respiratory failure (Chapter 20), where concomitant hypoxia can cause metabolic acidosis in addition to the primary respiratory acidosis. A useful diagnostic aid is the **Flenley nomogram** (Fig. 10e). Only one type of disturbance is likely if the patient's arterial pH and P_{CO_2} fall within a band (95% confidence limits).

11 Control of breathing I: neural mechanisms

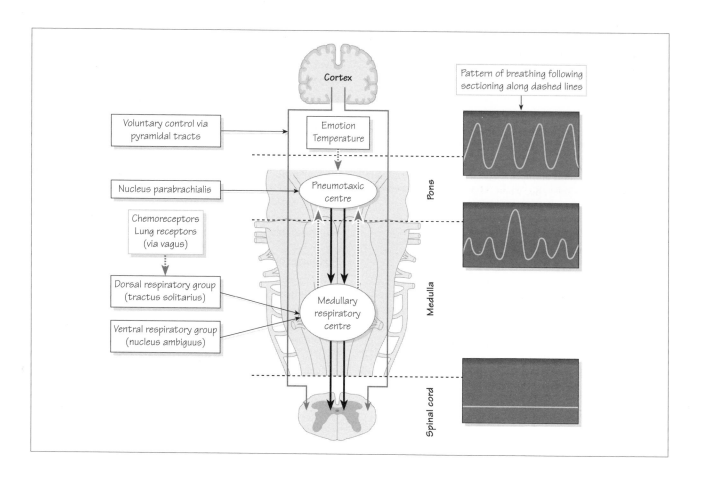

Control of breathing involves a **central controller** in the brainstem that sets the basic rhythm and pattern of ventilation and controls the **effectors** (respiratory muscles). It is modulated by higher centres and feedback from **sensors**, including the **chemoreceptors**, which match it to metabolism (Chapter 12) and **mechanoreceptors** in the lung (**lung receptors**). The neural networks involved are complex and not fully understood, reflecting the need to coordinate ventilation with functions such as coughing and vocalization.

Brainstem

The **pons** and **medulla** contain several diffuse groups of neurones that are associated with generation of the pattern and rhythm of breathing. Sectioning between the medulla and spinal cord abolishes breathing (Fig. 11). The **medullary respiratory centre** is located in the **reticular formation** of the ventrolateral medulla, beneath the floor of the 4th ventricle. This consists of a **dorsal respiratory group** in the **nucleus tractus solitarius**, containing inspiratory motor neurones leading to the respiratory muscles and a **ventral respiratory group** in and around the **nucleus ambiguus**, containing mainly expiratory neurones. There is **reciprocal innervation** between inspiratory and expiratory neurones, such that activity in one inhibits activity in the other. In eupnoea (normal breathing) expiration is passive and expiratory neurones show little activity. It is

thought the **pre-Bötzinger complex**, in the rostral part of the ventral respiratory group, forms the kernel of the **rhythm generator** for normal breathing, as neurones within it still exhibit cyclical firing when the complex is isolated from the rest of the brainstem.

The medullary respiratory centre is modulated by the **pneumotaxic centre**, located in the **nucleus parabrachialis** of the pons; sectioning between the pons and medulla alters the rhythm and pattern of breathing, but does not abolish it. The pneumotaxic centre receives both ascending input from the medullary respiratory centre and descending input from the hypothalamus and higher centres. Factors such as emotion and temperature affect breathing via this route, but the basic pattern of normal breathing is maintained following sectioning above the pons, although voluntary control is lost. Voluntary control of breathing is mediated by motor neurones from the cortex contained in the **pyramidal tract**, which bypasses both the pneumotaxic and medullary respiratory centres (Fig. 11). Certain rare lesions in the brainstem can therefore leave the voluntary pathways intact whilst impairing brainstem mechanisms, such that ventilation may cease when the patient falls asleep ('the curse of Ondine'). Some books refer to an **apneustic centre** in the lower pons, as sectioning here causes a characteristic gasping response. There is, however, little evidence that this is of physiological relevance.

The medullary respiratory centre receives ascending input through the tractus solitarius from the central and peripheral **chemoreceptors**, the latter via the **glossopharyngeal** nerve (Chapter 12) and from the **lung receptors** mainly via the **vagus**.

Lung receptors and reflexes

Stretch receptors: located in the smooth muscle of the bronchial walls. These are mostly **slowly adapting** (continue to fire with sustained stimulation), but there is a small rapidly adapting (transient) component. Their afferent nerves ascend via the vagus. Stimulation of stretch receptors causes breathing to be shorter and shallower and delays the next inspiratory cycle. These receptors are largely responsible for the **Hering–Breuer inspiratory reflex**, where lung inflation inhibits inspiratory muscle activity. Conversely, the **deflation reflex** augments inspiratory muscle activity on lung deflation. These reflexes are weak and unimportant during normal breathing in man, but are of more relevance when tidal volume is large (>1 L, e.g. in exercise) and in the neonate.

Juxtapulmonary or 'J' receptors: so called because they are located on the alveolar and bronchial walls, close to the capillaries. Their afferents are small unmyelinated (C-fibre) or myelinated nerves in the vagus. Activation causes apnoea (cessation of breathing) or rapid shallow breathing, falls in heart rate and blood pressure, laryngeal constriction and relaxation of skeletal muscles via spinal neurones. J receptors are stimulated by increased alveolar wall fluid, oedema, pulmonary congestion, microembolisms and inflammatory mediators such as histamine. All these stimuli are associated with many types of lung disease. The general action of J receptors is depression of somatic and visceral activity, which may be appropriate for serious lung damage.

Irritant receptors: located throughout airways between epithelial cells, with rapidly adapting afferent myelinated fibres in the vagus. Receptors in the trachea lead to cough; those in the lower airways lead to hyperpnoea. They also cause reflex bronchial and laryngeal constrictions. Irritant receptors are stimulated by irritant gases, smoke and dust (Chapters 17 and 31), but also by rapid large inflations and deflations, deformation of the airways, pulmonary congestion, inflammation and disease. Irritant receptors are responsible for the deep augmented breaths seen every 5–20 min at rest, which reverse the slow collapse of the lungs that occurs in quiet breathing. These receptors may be involved with first deep gasps of the newborn ('first breath') and are probably important for the Hering–Breuer deflationary reflex.

Proprioceptors (position/length sensors): located in the Golgi tendon organs, muscle spindles and joints of the respiratory muscles. Afferents lead to the spinal cord via the dorsal roots. Stimulated by shortening and load in respiratory muscles, though not diaphragm. They are important for coping with increased load and achieving optimal tidal volume and frequency. Note that input from non-respiratory muscles and joints can also stimulate breathing.

Other receptors that may modulate respiration:

Pain receptors: stimulation often causes brief apnoea followed by increased breathing.

Receptors in the *trigeminal region and larynx*: stimulation may give rise to apnoea or laryngeal spasm.

Arterial baroreceptors: stimulation depresses breathing.

12 Control of breathing II: chemical mechanisms

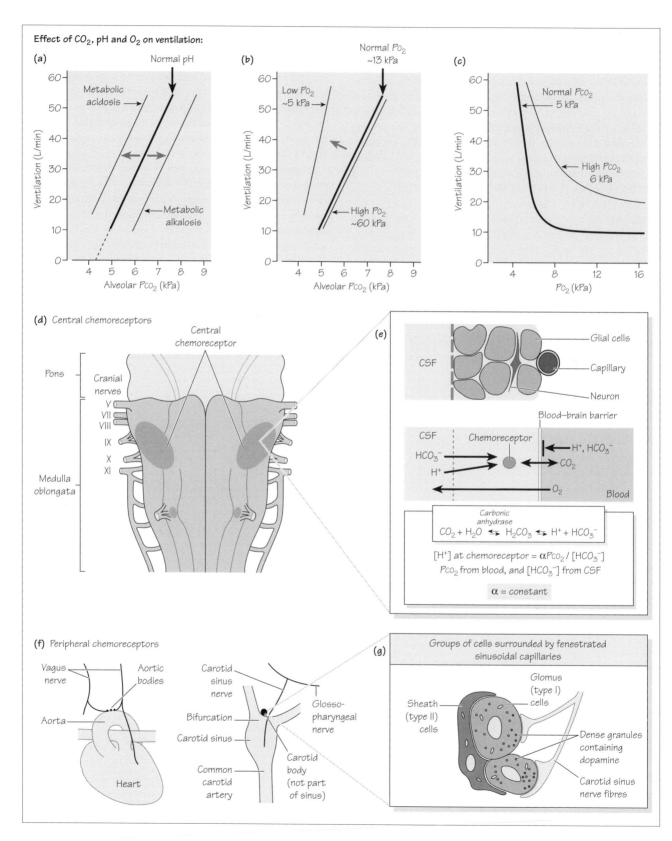

Effect of CO₂, pH and O₂ on ventilation:

(a) Ventilation (L/min) vs Alveolar P_{CO_2} (kPa). Normal pH. Metabolic acidosis. Metabolic alkalosis.

(b) Ventilation (L/min) vs Alveolar P_{CO_2} (kPa). Normal P_{O_2} ~13 kPa. Low P_{O_2} ~5 kPa. High P_{O_2} ~60 kPa.

(c) Ventilation (L/min) vs P_{O_2} (kPa). Normal P_{CO_2} 5 kPa. High P_{CO_2} 6 kPa.

(d) Central chemoreceptors. Central chemoreceptor. Pons. Cranial nerves. Medulla oblongata. V, VII, VIII, IX, X, XI.

(e) CSF. Glial cells. Capillary. Neuron. Blood–brain barrier. Chemoreceptor. HCO_3^-. H^+. H^+, HCO_3^-. CO_2. O_2. Blood.

Carbonic anhydrase
$$CO_2 + H_2O \rightleftharpoons H_2CO_3 \rightleftharpoons H^+ + HCO_3^-$$

$[H^+]$ at chemoreceptor $= \alpha P_{CO_2} / [HCO_3^-]$
P_{CO_2} from blood, and $[HCO_3^-]$ from CSF

$\alpha = $ constant

(f) Peripheral chemoreceptors. Vagus nerve. Aortic bodies. Aorta. Heart. Carotid sinus nerve. Glosso-pharyngeal nerve. Bifurcation. Carotid sinus. Common carotid artery. Carotid body (not part of sinus).

(g) Groups of cells surrounded by fenestrated sinusoidal capillaries. Glomus (type I) cells. Sheath (type II) cells. Dense granules containing dopamine. Carotid sinus nerve fibres.

Chemical control of ventilation is mediated via **chemoreceptors**, which detect arterial $P\text{CO}_2$, $P\text{O}_2$ and pH and modulate ventilation via the **respiratory centre** in the medulla (Chapter 11). $P\text{CO}_2$ is the most important factor. Ventilation is thus closely matched to metabolism—large changes in metabolic rate result in very small changes in arterial $P\text{CO}_2$ and $P\text{O}_2$.

Normal alveolar $P\text{CO}_2$ ($P_A\text{CO}_2$) is ~5.3 kPa (40 mmHg). Increasing $P_A\text{CO}_2$ causes minute ventilation (litres ventilated per minute) to rise in an almost linear fashion (Fig. 12a), by ~15–25 L/min for each kPa rise in $P_A\text{CO}_2$ (~2.7 L/min/mmHg). There is considerable variation between individuals, and athletes and patients with chronic respiratory disease often have a reduced response to $P_A\text{CO}_2$ (Chapters 24 and 40). If $P_A\text{CO}_2$ increases above 10 kPa, ventilation decreases due to direct suppression of the respiratory centre. A **metabolic acidosis** (an increase in [H+] caused by reduced [HCO_3^-]; see Chapter 10) shifts the CO_2–ventilation response curve to the left, whereas a **metabolic alkalosis** shifts it to the right (Fig. 12a). Note that a rise in [H+] caused by increased $P\text{CO}_2$ is called a **respiratory acidosis**. Increasing $P_A\text{O}_2$ from the normal value of ~13 kPa (~100 mmHg) has little effect on the CO_2–ventilation response curve, but if the $P_A\text{O}_2$ is reduced, the slope of the relationship becomes steeper and ventilation increases more for any given rise in $P_A\text{CO}_2$ (Fig. 12b). When the effect of $P_A\text{O}_2$ is investigated independently (at constant $P_A\text{CO}_2$), there is little increase in ventilation until the $P_A\text{O}_2$ falls below ~8 kPa (~60 mmHg) (Fig. 12c). The effect of reducing $P_A\text{O}_2$ is, however, potentiated if the $P_A\text{CO}_2$ is raised—i.e. there is a **synergistic** (more than additive) relationship between the effects of $P_A\text{O}_2$ and $P_A\text{CO}_2$.

The chemoreceptors

The **central chemoreceptor** consists of a diffuse collection of neurones located near the ventrolateral surface of the medulla, close to the exit of the 9th and 10th cranial nerves (Fig. 12d). It is sensitive to the pH of the surrounding cerebrospinal fluid (CSF) and does **not** respond to $P\text{O}_2$. CSF is separated from blood by the **blood–brain barrier**, a tight endothelial layer lining the blood vessels of the brain. This barrier is impermeable to polar molecules such as H+ and HCO_3^-, but CO_2 can diffuse across it easily. The pH of CSF is therefore determined by the arterial $P\text{CO}_2$ and the CSF [HCO_3^-] (Chapter 10) and is not directly affected by changes in blood pH (Fig. 12e). CSF contains little protein, so its buffering capacity is low; therefore a small change in $P\text{CO}_2$ will cause a large change in pH. Stimulation of the central chemoreceptor by a fall in CSF pH (rise in blood $P\text{CO}_2$) causes an increase in ventilation. The central chemoreceptor is responsible for ~80% of the response to CO_2 in humans. It has a relatively slow response time (~20 s), as CO_2 has to diffuse across the blood–brain barrier.

The **peripheral chemoreceptors** are the **carotid** and **aortic bodies**. The carotid body is a small (~2 mg) structure located at the bifurcation of the common carotid artery, just above the carotid sinus. It is innervated by the carotid sinus nerve, leading to the glossopharyngeal (Fig. 12f). The aortic bodies are found on the aortic arch and are innervated by the vagus. In humans, they are less important than carotid bodies. The carotid body contains **glomus** (type I) cells and **sheath** (type II) cells (Fig. 12g). Glomus cells are responsible for chemoreception; they have dense granules containing dopamine and contact axons of the carotid sinus nerve. The function of sheath cells is unclear.

Carotid bodies respond to increased $P\text{CO}_2$ or [H+] and decreased $P\text{O}_2$ (**not** blood O_2 content) by increasing firing rate in the carotid sinus nerve, and thus ventilation. They have a high blood flow and consequently a small arteriovenous difference for $P\text{CO}_2$ and $P\text{O}_2$. They respond rapidly (seconds) and are sufficiently fast to detect small oscillations in blood gases associated with breathing. The mechanisms by which changes in $P\text{CO}_2$, pH and $P\text{O}_2$ are detected are unclear, but for $P\text{O}_2$ they are believed to involve inhibition of K+ channels in the glomus cell, with consequent depolarization and Ca^{2+} entry.

Adaptation: chronic respiratory disease and altitude

When hypercapnia (raised arterial $P\text{CO}_2$) is prolonged, for example in chronic respiratory disease, CSF pH gradually returns to normal due to an adaptive increase in HCO_3^- transport across the blood–brain barrier. The drive to breathe from the central chemoreceptor is consequently reduced, even though $P\text{CO}_2$ is still high. Associated with this, there is occasionally a loss of sensitivity to further increases in $P_a\text{CO}_2$, and the patient's ventilation is then primarily controlled by the level of $P\text{O}_2$ (**hypoxic drive**). Care must be taken with such patients, as giving high concentrations of O_2 in order to increase blood O_2 saturation may raise the $P\text{O}_2$ sufficiently to depress the hypoxic drive and hence ventilation. Normally, ~24–28% O_2 is given to such patients. This leads to a sufficiently small rise in $P_a\text{CO}_2$ as to have little effect on the hypoxic drive, but because of the steep slope of the O_2 dissociation curve (Chapter 8) it can result in a significant improvement in O_2 content.

At high altitudes, ventilation is stimulated by the low atmospheric $P\text{O}_2$. This leads to **hypocapnia** and alkalosis (as CO_2 is blown off), which depress ventilation. Over some days, the pH of CSF returns to normal due to HCO_3^- transport out of the CSF, even though the $P\text{CO}_2$ remains low and ventilation increases again. Over a longer period blood pH returns to normal due to renal compensation (Chapter 10). These processes form part of the acclimatization to altitude.

13 Pulmonary circulation and anatomical right-to-left shunts

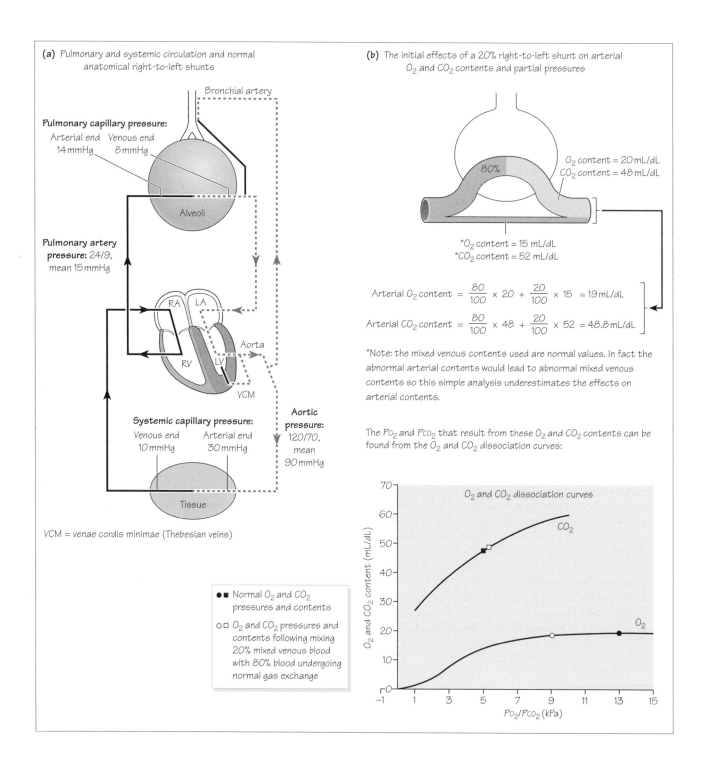

(a) Pulmonary and systemic circulation and normal anatomical right-to-left shunts

Pulmonary capillary pressure:
Arterial end 14 mmHg   Venous end 8 mmHg

Bronchial artery

Alveoli

Pulmonary artery pressure: 24/9, mean 15 mmHg

RA   LA

Aorta

RV   LV

VCM

Systemic capillary pressure:
Venous end 10 mmHg   Arterial end 30 mmHg

Aortic pressure: 120/70, mean 90 mmHg

Tissue

VCM = venae cordis minimae (Thebesian veins)

● ■ Normal O_2 and CO_2 pressures and contents

○ □ O_2 and CO_2 pressures and contents following mixing 20% mixed venous blood with 80% blood undergoing normal gas exchange

(b) The initial effects of a 20% right-to-left shunt on arterial O_2 and CO_2 contents and partial pressures

80%

O_2 content = 20 mL/dL
CO_2 content = 48 mL/dL

*O_2 content = 15 mL/dL
*CO_2 content = 52 mL/dL

$$\text{Arterial } O_2 \text{ content} = \frac{80}{100} \times 20 + \frac{20}{100} \times 15 = 19\,\text{mL/dL}$$

$$\text{Arterial } CO_2 \text{ content} = \frac{80}{100} \times 48 + \frac{20}{100} \times 52 = 48.8\,\text{mL/dL}$$

*Note: the mixed venous contents used are normal values. In fact the abnormal arterial contents would lead to abnormal mixed venous contents so this simple analysis underestimates the effects on arterial contents.

The Po_2 and Pco_2 that result from these O_2 and CO_2 contents can be found from the O_2 and CO_2 dissociation curves:

O_2 and CO_2 dissociation curves

CO_2

O_2

O_2 and CO_2 content (mL/dL)

Po_2/Pco_2 (kPa)

Pulmonary circulation compared with the systemic circulation (Fig. 13a)

The **pulmonary circulation** is in series with the **systemic circulation** and pulmonary blood flow nearly equals aortic blood flow. **Pulmonary vascular resistance** is only about one-sixth of systemic resistance and the thin-walled right ventricle need only generate a mean **pulmonary artery pressure** of about 15 mmHg to drive the cardiac output through the lungs. Systemic pressures are higher (Fig. 13a), dropping steeply across the main resistance vessel, the arteriole, to give a capillary flow which is usually non-pulsatile.

Pulmonary vascular resistance is more evenly distributed in the microcirculation and pulmonary capillary flow remains pulsatile.

Local systemic resistance and blood flow are controlled by sympathetic nerves, metabolites and other substances acting on arterioles. Both sympathetic and parasympathetic nerves innervate pulmonary vessels, but their influence is weak in most circumstances. Systemic arterioles dilate in response to hypoxia, increasing flow and hence oxygen delivery. In contrast, **hypoxic vasoconstriction** occurs in the pulmonary circulation. This response, which is accentuated by high P_{CO_2}, improves gas exchange by diverting blood from underventilated to well-ventilated regions (Chapter 14). The response is unhelpful in the presence of global lung hypoxia, at altitude or in respiratory failure, where it may contribute to the development of pulmonary hypertension and right heart failure.

As cardiac output increases in exercise, pulmonary vascular resistance falls, as vessels are recruited and distended and the rise in pulmonary arterial pressure is small. The pulmonary circulation acts as a blood reservoir and the volume it contains varies, being about 450 mL when upright and 800 mL lying down. Inspiration also increases pulmonary vascular volume.

Fluid balance across capillaries is determined by hydrostatic and oncotic pressures (the **Starling forces**; see *The Cardiovascular System at a Glance*, Chapter 20) across capillary walls. **Capillary oncotic pressure** opposes filtration and is about 27 mmHg in both circulations. Although hydrostatic pressure is low in the pulmonary capillaries (about 10 mmHg), net filtration of fluid occurs in pulmonary capillaries as it does in systemic capillaries. Other factors favouring filtration are **interstitial oncotic pressure**, which is relatively high in the lungs (about 18 mmHg) and **interstitial hydrostatic pressure**, which is negative (about –4 mmHg). **Pulmonary oedema** occurs when these forces are altered to increase net filtration above the rate that can be cleared by the pulmonary lymphatics. For example, it may occur when pulmonary capillary pressure is increased in **mitral stenosis** and **left ventricular failure**. **Inspiratory crepitations** (crackles) on auscultation in these conditions are probably caused by popping open of airways in lungs stiffened by congestion with blood. They are most obvious at the bases, where hydrostatic pressure is highest. Pulmonary congestion and oedema are worsened by the increase in pulmonary blood volume lying down.

Anatomical or true right-to-left shunts

Ideally, all venous blood emerging from tissues would return to the right side of the heart to be pumped through gas-exchanging lung. In fact, part of the blood draining the **bronchial circulation** joins the pulmonary vein. This part results in deoxygenated blood from the airways contaminating blood returning from alveoli (Fig. 13a). In addition, a small amount of the coronary venous blood drains directly into the left ventricular cavity via the **venae cordis minimae (Thebesian veins)**. These additions of deoxygenated (right-sided) blood to oxygenated (left-sided) blood are known as anatomical **right-to-left shunts**. In normal people, they are equivalent to 2% or less of the cardiac output, but they explain why arterial P_{O_2} is less than alveolar P_{O_2} even though pulmonary capillary blood equilibrates with alveolar gas.

In disease, right-to-left shunting of blood may be much larger. **Atelectasis** (lung collapse) or **consolidation** in **pneumonia** will result in pulmonary arterial blood supplying the affected region failing to undergo gas exchange. Right-to-left shunts are also the cause of reduced arterial oxygenation in **cyanotic congenital heart disease** such as **tetralogy of Fallot**. Atrial or ventricular septal defects do not usually cause impaired gas exchange and cyanosis, as the higher left-sided pressures give rise to **left-to-right shunts** in which some oxygenated blood is pumped again through the lungs.

The effect of right-to-left shunts on arterial blood gases

In the right-to-left shunt shown schematically in Fig. 13b, 20% of blood fails to pass through functioning alveoli and its O_2 and CO_2 contents remain at mixed venous levels of 15 and 52 mL/dL, respectively. Eighty per cent of the blood undergoes normal gas exchange, emerging with normal O_2 and CO_2 contents of 20 and 48 mL/dL, respectively. The initial effect on arterial gas contents is calculated from a weighted average of the contents in these two blood streams. This gives an arterial O_2 content 1 mL/dL below normal and CO_2 content 0.8 mL/dL above normal. From the flat part of the oxygen dissociation curve, it can be seen that the resulting arterial P_{O_2} is about 9 kPa (68 mmHg) compared with the normal 13 kPa (97 mmHg). The much steeper CO_2 dissociation curve means the rise in P_{CO_2} is small, from the normal value of 5.3 kPa (40 mmHg) to about 5.5 kPa (41 mmHg).

If the respiratory system is otherwise normal, the reduced P_aO_2 and increased P_aCO_2 simulate ventilation via the chemoreceptors and CO_2 washed out of the functioning areas restores arterial CO_2 content and P_aCO_2 to normal. In contrast, increased ventilation has little effect on arterial oxygen content and P_{O_2}, as blood draining the ventilated areas of the lung was already saturated. If hypoxia is severe, the stimulation in ventilation is often great enough to reduce P_aCO_2 below normal. Typically, in a right-to-left shunt there is a low P_aO_2 with a normal or low P_aCO_2.

14 Ventilation–perfusion mismatching

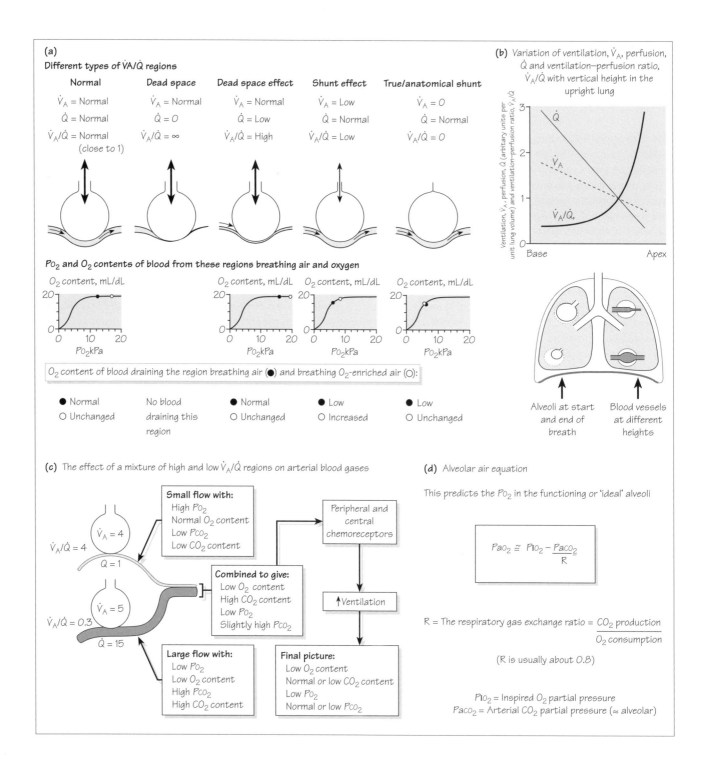

(a)
Different types of $\dot{V}A/\dot{Q}$ regions

Normal	Dead space	Dead space effect	Shunt effect	True/anatomical shunt
$\dot{V}_A$ = Normal	$\dot{V}_A$ = Normal	$\dot{V}_A$ = Normal	$\dot{V}_A$ = Low	$\dot{V}_A$ = 0
$\dot{Q}$ = Normal	$\dot{Q}$ = 0	$\dot{Q}$ = Low	$\dot{Q}$ = Normal	$\dot{Q}$ = Normal
$\dot{V}_A/\dot{Q}$ = Normal (close to 1)	$\dot{V}_A/\dot{Q}$ = ∞	$\dot{V}_A/\dot{Q}$ = High	$\dot{V}_A/\dot{Q}$ = Low	$\dot{V}_A/\dot{Q}$ = 0

(b) Variation of ventilation, $\dot{V}_A$, perfusion, $\dot{Q}$ and ventilation–perfusion ratio, $\dot{V}_A/\dot{Q}$ with vertical height in the upright lung

Po_2 and O_2 contents of blood from these regions breathing air and oxygen

O_2 content, mL/dL

O_2 content of blood draining the region breathing air (●) and breathing O_2-enriched air (○):

- ● Normal
- ○ Unchanged

No blood draining this region

- ● Normal
- ○ Unchanged

- ● Low
- ○ Increased

- ● Low
- ○ Unchanged

Alveoli at start and end of breath

Blood vessels at different heights

(c) The effect of a mixture of high and low $\dot{V}_A/\dot{Q}$ regions on arterial blood gases

$\dot{V}_A/\dot{Q}$ = 4 $\dot{V}_A$ = 4   Q = 1

Small flow with:
High Po_2
Normal O_2 content
Low Pco_2
Low CO_2 content

Peripheral and central chemoreceptors

Combined to give:
Low O_2 content
High CO_2 content
Low Po_2
Slightly high Pco_2

↑Ventilation

$\dot{V}_A/\dot{Q}$ = 0.3 $\dot{V}_A$ = 5 $\dot{Q}$ = 15

Large flow with:
Low Po_2
Low O_2 content
High Pco_2
High CO_2 content

Final picture:
Low O_2 content
Normal or low CO_2 content
Low Po_2
Normal or low Pco_2

(d) Alveolar air equation

This predicts the Po_2 in the functioning or 'ideal' alveoli

$$Pao_2 \cong Pio_2 - \frac{Paco_2}{R}$$

R = The respiratory gas exchange ratio = $\dfrac{CO_2 \text{ production}}{O_2 \text{ consumption}}$

(R is usually about 0.8)

Pio_2 = Inspired O_2 partial pressure
$Paco_2$ = Arterial CO_2 partial pressure (≈ alveolar)

At rest, alveolar ventilation and pulmonary blood flow are similar, each being around 5 L/min. Ventilation (V_A) and perfusion (Q) may vary in different lung regions, but for optimal gas exchange they must be matched. Areas with high perfusion need high ventilation and ideally, local ventilation–perfusion ratios (V_A/Q) should be close to 1. Ventilation–perfusion mismatching or inequality is said to occur when regional V_A/Q ratios vary, with many being much greater or less than 1 (Fig. 14a). A right-to-left shunt from complete collapse or consolidation of a region (Chapter 13) has $V_A/Q = 0$, and can be viewed as an extreme example of ventilation–perfusion mismatching. At the other extreme, alveolar dead space from a pulmonary embolus is a ventilated region without perfusion and $V_A/Q = \infty$. Regions where V_A/Q is much greater than 1 have excessive ventilation or **dead space effect** and blood from them has a high P_{O_2} and a low P_{CO_2}. Regions with V_A/Q much less than 1 behave qualitatively like shunts and are sources of **shunt effect** or **venous admixture**. Blood draining them has undergone some gas exchange, but P_{O_2} is lower and P_{CO_2} higher than normal. The effect on P_{O_2} and O_2 content draining different V_A/Q regions both during air breathing and during oxygen breathing is shown in Fig. 14a (lower panel).

Effect of the upright posture on perfusion, ventilation and V_A/Q (Fig. 14b)

Hydrostatic pressure in all vessels varies with vertical height above or below the heart, because of the weight of blood. On standing, the increased pressure at the lung bases distends vessels, increasing flow. Pressures generated by the right heart are low and higher up the lung vascular pressures in diastole may fall below alveolar pressure at the venous end of the pulmonary capillary. In such regions, flow is reduced and determined by the difference between arterial and alveolar pressure. There may be regions at the apices—especially in haemorrhage or positive-pressure breathing—where alveolar pressure also exceeds pressure at the arterial end of the pulmonary capillaries. The vessels collapse completely for part of each cardiac cycle, giving low, intermittent flow. The net result is a blood flow per unit volume of lung tissue that falls progressively from base to apex.

Gravity also affects intrapleural pressure, which is less negative at the base than the apex. As a result, at functional residual capacity apical alveoli are more expanded—with less capacity for further expansion during inspiration—than at the bases. Consequently, ventilation is also higher at the base than the apex. The effect of gravity on ventilation is less marked than on perfusion and so V_A/Q is higher at the apex than the base. In young people, this modest degree of mismatching has little effect on blood gases. The scatter of ventilation–perfusion ratios increases with age and contributes to the reduction in P_aO_2 seen in the elderly.

Ventilation–perfusion matching in disease

Increased ventilation–perfusion mismatching is an important cause of gas exchange problems in many respiratory diseases, including asthma, chronic obstructive pulmonary disease (COPD), pneumonia and pulmonary oedema. Regions of low V_A/Q may arise when airways are partly blocked by bronchoconstriction, inflammation or secretions and high V_A/Q in emphysematous areas where capillaries are lost. **Hypoxic vasoconstriction** (Chapter 13) helps reduce the severity of ventilation–perfusion mismatching.

Effect of ventilation–perfusion mismatching on arterial blood gases

Blood emerging from areas with high V_A/Q might be expected to compensate for blood from areas with low V_A/Q. This is not the case, for two reasons (Fig. 14c). Firstly, although P_{O_2} will be increased in high V_A/Q regions, oxygen content is raised little, as blood is normally nearly saturated. Blood draining regions with low V_A/Q and low P_{O_2} (especially if <8 kPa, 60 mmHg) will have significantly reduced oxygen content. In addition, these areas contribute more blood than areas with high V_A/Q, which are typically caused by reduced perfusion. The net effect of mixing blood from areas with a wide range of ventilation–perfusion ratios is a low arterial O_2 content and P_aO_2. CO_2 content is less severely affected because the overventilated areas do lose extra CO_2 and partly compensate for low V_A/Q regions. Moreover, any abnormalities of P_aO_2 and P_aCO_2 will lead to a reflex increase in ventilation, which usually corrects or overcorrects the raised P_aCO_2 whilst being less effective at raising P_aO_2. The final arterial blood gas picture, a low P_aO_2 and a normal or low P_aCO_2, is similar to that resulting from anatomical right-to-left shunts (Chapter 13).

One difference is that arterial hypoxia caused by ventilation–perfusion mismatching improves much more with oxygen therapy than that caused by a shunt. In shunts, the **oxygen-enriched air** fails to reach the shunted blood. In V_A/Q mismatching, increased oxygen fraction can increase local P_{O_2} in areas of low V_A/Q (Fig. 14a), giving rise to significant improvement in arterial oxygen content and pressure.

Assessment of ventilation–perfusion mismatching

Regional ventilation and perfusion can be visualized by inhalation and infusion of appropriate radioisotopes (Chapter 19). A simple but useful index of the degree of mismatching is the difference between P_{O_2} in gas-exchanging or 'ideal' alveoli and in arterial blood. Ideal alveolar P_{O_2} can be calculated from the **alveolar air equation** (Fig. 14d). An increased **A–a P_{O_2} gradient** (A = alveolar P_{O_2}, a = arterial P_{O_2}) is usually caused by ventilation–perfusion mismatching or anatomical right-to-left shunts. In normal young people, there is a small A–a gradient (<2 kPa) arising from the normal anatomical right-to-left shunts discussed in Chapter 13.

15 Development of the respiratory system and birth

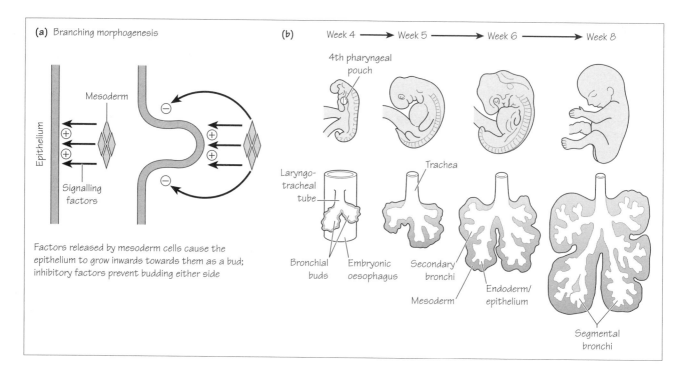

(a) Branching morphogenesis

Factors released by mesoderm cells cause the epithelium to grow inwards towards them as a bud; inhibitory factors prevent budding either side

(b) Week 4 ⟶ Week 5 ⟶ Week 6 ⟶ Week 8

The **embryological origins** of the lung are primitive **endoderm** of the foregut, which eventually forms the epithelium and glands of the larynx, trachea and lungs and **splanchnic mesoderm**, which forms cartilage, smooth muscle, lung parenchyma and connective tissue. In common with many glandular organs, the lung develops by **branching morphogenesis** (Fig. 15a), with budding and branching of the endoderm/epithelium into mesoderm. The process requires reciprocal signalling between epithelium and mesoderm, with the mesoderm being primarily responsible for programming development of adjacent epithelium into the relevant structures. Many signalling molecules are vital for the orchestration of branching morphogenesis during lung development, including fibroblast growth factors (FGF), epidermal growth factor (EGF), bone morphogenetic proteins and sonic hedgehog. Development of the respiratory system is generally divided into five stages or periods.

Embryonic period: the tracheobronchial tree originates from the **laryngotracheal tube**, below the 4th pharyngeal pouch at the caudal (tail) end of the primordial pharynx. The laryngotracheal tube starts to appear just prior to the 4th week of development, after the heart begins to beat. By the end of the 4th week, its end has bifurcated into two **bronchial buds**, progenitors of the two main bronchi and bronchial tree (Fig. 15b).

Pseudoglandular period (5th–17th weeks): the bronchial buds have now developed into the primordial left and (slightly larger) right primary bronchi, which subsequently divide by branching morphogenesis into five secondary bronchi (three right, two left). At the 7th week, these have started to branch progressively into 10 (right) or eight to nine (left) **segmental** (tertiary) bronchi, each of which eventually forms a **bronchopulmonary segment**. By the

17th week, most of the major structures of the lung have formed and are lined with glycogen-rich columnar epithelial cells. The gas exchange surfaces have not yet developed and fetuses delivered during this period are therefore not viable.

Canalicular period (16th–25th weeks): bronchial cartilage, smooth muscle, abundant pulmonary capillaries and connective tissue develop from the mesoderm. There is progressive differentiation and thinning of epithelial cells. The bronchi will have subdivided ~17 times after 24 weeks, finally forming the respiratory bronchioles which themselves divide into three to six alveolar ducts and some thin-walled **terminal sacs**. These are lined by very thin **type I alveolar pneumocytes** (squamous epithelium), which together with endothelial cells from capillaries form the future **alveolacapillary membrane** (gas exchange surface). There are a few **type II alveolar pneumocytes**, secretory epithelial cells that produce surfactant. This reduces surface tension and allows expansion of the terminal sacs/alveoli (Chapter 6), but although it is present in small amounts from about the 20th week, there is insufficient to support unaided breathing until after 26 weeks (see **neonatal respiratory distress syndrome**, Chapter 16). Some gas exchange can occur at the end of this period, as there are both thin-walled terminal sacs and good vascularization, but the general level of immaturity means that fetuses born before the end of the 24th week normally die despite intensive care.

Saccular (terminal sac) period (24th week–parturition): associated with rapid development in the number of terminal sacs and the pulmonary and lymphatic capillary networks. Budding from the terminal sacs and walls of terminal bronchioles and thinning of type I pneumocytes leads to formation of immature alveoli from around week 32. Sufficient surfactant and vascularization are normally present between the 24th and 26th week to allow survival of some premature fetuses, though this is very variable (see Chapter 16). Surfactant increases significantly in the two weeks before birth.

Alveolar period (late fetal to childhood): clusters of immature alveoli form during the early part of this period; mature-type alveoli do not appear until after birth. **Fetal breathing** movements are present before birth, with aspiration of amniotic fluid, and these stimulate lung growth and respiratory muscle conditioning. Lung development is impaired in the absence of fetal breathing, inadequate amniotic fluid (**oligohydramnios**) or space for lung growth (see Chapter 16). The increase in lung size over the first 3 years is due primarily to an increase in number of alveoli and respiratory bronchioles; thereafter, both the number and size of alveoli increase. More than 90% of alveoli are formed after birth, reaching a maximum after 7–8 years. At the end of lung development, there are approximately 23 generations of airways, with ~17 million branches.

Birth

The lungs are initially 50% full of fluid at birth, which is replaced by air. During and immediately following birth, fluid is removed via the pulmonary and lymphatic circulations and through the mouth as a result of squeezing during delivery. Expansion and filling of the alveoli with air is critically dependent on the presence of surfactant to lower surface tension. Before birth, the vascular resistance of the pulmonary circulation is higher than that of the systemic and blood is consequently shunted via the ductus arteriosus and foramen ovale (see *The Cardiovascular System at a Glance,* Chapter 25). At birth, the increased arterial P_{O_2} rapidly reduces the pulmonary vascular resistance below that of the systemic and constricts the ductus arteriosus. Blood therefore starts to flow through the lungs, the pressure gradient across the foramen ovale reverses, causing closure, and blood flow takes its adult course.

16 Complications of development and congenital disease

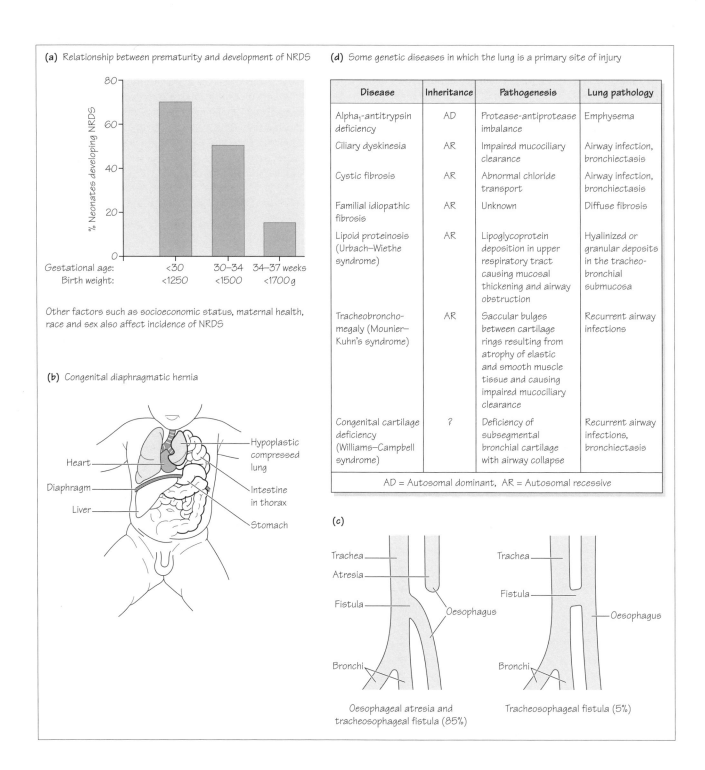

(a) Relationship between prematurity and development of NRDS

% Neonates developing NRDS

Gestational age: <30 30–34 34–37 weeks
Birth weight: <1250 <1500 <1700 g

Other factors such as socioeconomic status, maternal health, race and sex also affect incidence of NRDS

(b) Congenital diaphragmatic hernia

Heart
Diaphragm
Liver

Hypoplastic compressed lung
Intestine in thorax
Stomach

(d) Some genetic diseases in which the lung is a primary site of injury

Disease	Inheritance	Pathogenesis	Lung pathology
Alpha₁-antitrypsin deficiency	AD	Protease-antiprotease imbalance	Emphysema
Ciliary dyskinesia	AR	Impaired mucociliary clearance	Airway infection, bronchiectasis
Cystic fibrosis	AR	Abnormal chloride transport	Airway infection, bronchiectasis
Familial idiopathic fibrosis	AR	Unknown	Diffuse fibrosis
Lipoid proteinosis (Urbach–Wiethe syndrome)	AR	Lipoglycoprotein deposition in upper respiratory tract causing mucosal thickening and airway obstruction	Hyalinized or granular deposits in the tracheo-bronchial submucosa
Tracheobroncho-megaly (Mounier–Kuhn's syndrome)	AR	Saccular bulges between cartilage rings resulting from atrophy of elastic and smooth muscle tissue and causing impaired mucociliary clearance	Recurrent airway infections
Congenital cartilage deficiency (Williams–Campbell syndrome)	?	Deficiency of subsegmental bronchial cartilage with airway collapse	Recurrent airway infections, bronchiectasis
AD = Autosomal dominant, AR = Autosomal recessive			

(c)

Trachea
Atresia
Fistula
Oesophagus
Bronchi

Oesophageal atresia and tracheosophageal fistula (85%)

Trachea
Fistula
Oesophagus
Bronchi

Tracheosophageal fistula (5%)

Problems associated with premature birth

Neonatal respiratory distress syndrome (NRDS), otherwise known as hyaline membrane disease, occurs in ~2% of all births and is characterized by rapid, laboured breathing and often sternal retraction due to partial collapse of the lungs after each breath. Lung compliance is low. NRDS is most commonly caused by lack of sufficient quantities of surfactant and consequent high surface tension in the alveoli and small airways. Incidence therefore increases sharply with degree of prematurity (Fig. 16a), although other factors may also reduce production of surfactant. When a premature birth is anticipated, the expectant mother can be treated with **corticosteroids** (betamethasone) to speed fetal lung development and surfactant production. Treatment with **exogenous surfactant** in the first 30 min after birth, either of natural origin or artificial, has also proved to be beneficial. Survival of neonates with NRDS often requires high positive pressure mechanical ventilation and high levels of oxygen.

The large majority of NRDS cases are related to prematurity, with some due to other causes including damage to type II pneumocytes. A very few cases are due to a congenital absence of **pulmonary surfactant protein B**. These patients do not respond to any form of therapy and tend to die in the first few months of life.

Bronchopulmonary dysplasia (chronic lung disease of the newborn) is a long-term consequence of NRDS, primarily as a result of treatment with high positive pressure ventilation combined with high levels of oxygen (hyperoxia). The condition is characterized by alterations in the structure and function of airways and pulmonary blood vessels, including increases in airway and vascular smooth muscle and obliteration of some microstructures. This leads to poorly reversible airway obstruction and sometimes pulmonary hypertension (high pulmonary blood pressure). Survivors may retain symptoms for many years, if not for life. There are several similarities to chronic obstructive pulmonary disease (COPD, Chapter 23) and chronic severe asthma in adults.

Several techniques have recently been designed to minimize the incidence of bronchopulmonary dysplasia in infants with NRDS. These include extracorporeal membrane oxygenation (**ECMO**), where blood is circulated via external apparatus for gas exchange; mechanical ventilation and hyperoxia are therefore not required and some success has been reported. Conversely, ECMO has not been found useful in adults with acute respiratory distress syndrome (ARDS, Chapter 35). **Partial fluid ventilation**, where the lungs are ventilated with fluids containing oxygen-carrying perfluorocarbons, has also been reported to be beneficial. Fluid ventilation circumvents problems associated with high surface tension by removing the air–liquid interface and allows small airways to open and contribute to gas exchange.

Congenital diseases

Congenital diaphragmatic hernia is the most common cause of lung hypoplasia (inadequate development of the lung), with an incidence of about one in 2000 births. Failure of the diaphragm to fuse with the membranes on the thoracic and peritoneal wall leads to a posterolateral defect, most commonly occurring on the left side (~85%), through which the abdominal viscera pass (herniate) into the thorax (Fig. 16b). This often includes the stomach, spleen and much of the intestines. The presence of the resultant mass severely restricts lung development and later inflation, leading to a significantly reduced lung volume and life-threatening breathing difficulties. The latter are the prime cause of death in congenital diaphragmatic hernia and most infants will die because the lungs are insufficiently developed to support life outside the uterus. Although surgical correction of the defect is possible both before and after birth, the mortality rate is very high. A related but very much less common condition is **eventration of the diaphragm**, where half the diaphragm lacks adequate muscle and bulges (eventrates) into the thoracic cavity. The viscera are forced into the pocket so formed, again restricting lung development.

Tracheoesophageal fistula (an opening between oesophagus and trachea) is the most common abnormality of the lower respiratory tract itself, with an incidence of about one in 4000 births. Its origins are located in the 4th week of development, when the embryonic respiratory tract starts to develop and divide from the embryonic oesophagus (see Chapter 15). Eighty-five per cent of cases are associated with the descending part of the oesophagus having a blind ending (**oesophageal atresia**) (Fig. 16c); the lower part of the oesophagus joins instead to the base of the trachea. As a result, normal feeding is impossible and the gut becomes distended with air. There are also consequences *in utero*, as normally amniotic fluid is ingested by the fetus. Thus oesophageal atresia is commonly associated with excess amniotic fluid (**polyhydramnios**), which can lead to severe defects in the central nervous system. Some 5% of cases of tracheoesophageal fistula show no atresia but only a fistula, and the remainder less common variations. Rare defects involving blockage or narrowing of the trachea itself (**tracheal atresia/stenosis**) are nearly always accompanied by various types of tracheoesophageal fistula.

Congenital influences on respiratory disease: several important respiratory diseases that are discussed in detail in other chapters have definite or implied genetic components, including asthma (Chapter 21), chronic obstructive pulmonary disease (Chapter 23), emphysema (Chapter 23), cystic fibrosis (Chapter 30) and primary pulmonary hypertension (Chapter 24). Other genetically linked diseases that cause pathological problems primarily in the lung are listed in Fig. 16d.

17 Lung defence mechanisms and immunology

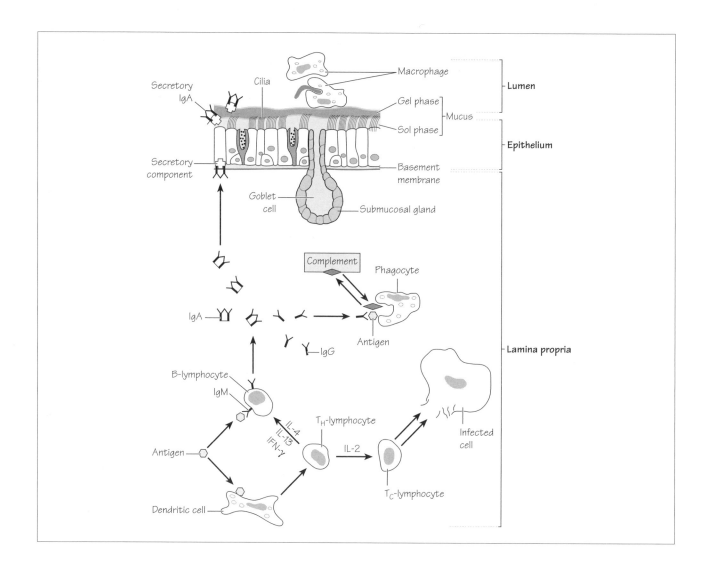

Inhalation of air also allows ingress of dust, irritant particles and pathogens. The huge surface area of the lungs provides multiple opportunities for damage, and the warm, humid environment provides ideal conditions for bacterial and other infestations. The respiratory tract, however, has a range of powerful defence mechanisms. Dysfunction of these mechanisms underlies many respiratory diseases, for example asthma (Chapter 21) and fibrosis (Chapters 27 and 31).

Physical and physiological defences

The nostrils and nasopharynx provide a physical barrier to particles >10 μm, in the form of hairs and mucus to which particles adhere. **Mucociliary transport** (see below) subsequently transfers these to the pharynx, where they are ingested. Only particles less than 5 μm generally get further than the trachea. The nasopharynx also provides important **humidifying** and **warming** functions for inhaled air, preventing drying of epithelium. Irritant particles in the nose

and trachea, whether inhaled or transported from distal regions by mucociliary transport, stimulate irritant receptors (Chapter 11), provoking sneezing and coughing that eject foreign matter.

Mucus and airway secretions

The respiratory epithelium is covered with a 5–10 μm layer of gelatinous mucus (gel phase) floating on a slightly thinner fluid layer (sol phase) (Fig. 17). The **cilia** on epithelial cells beat synchronously, and as they do so their tips catch in the gel phase and cause it to move towards the mouth, transporting particles and cellular debris with it (mucociliary transport or clearance). It takes ~40 min for mucus from large bronchi to reach the pharynx and from respiratory bronchioles several days. Many factors can disrupt this mechanism, including an increase in mucus viscosity or thickness, making it harder to move (e.g. inflammation, asthma), changes in the sol phase that inhibit cilia movement or prevent attachment to the gel phase and defects in cilia activity (**cilia dyskinaesia**). Mucociliary transport is reduced by smoking, pollutants, anaesthetics and infection, and in **cystic fibrosis** (Chapter 30) and the rare congenital immotile cilia syndrome. Reduced mucociliary transport causes recurrent respiratory infections that progressively damage the lungs—for example, **bronchiectasis**, where the bronchial walls are thickened, permanently dilated and inflamed (see Chapters 30 and 40).

Mucus is produced by **goblet cells** in the epithelium and **submucosal glands**. The major constituents are carbohydrate-rich glycoproteins called mucins that give mucus its gel-like nature. The fluidity and ionic composition of the sol phase is controlled by epithelial cells. Mucus contains several factors produced by epithelial and other cells or derived from plasma: **anti-proteases** such as α_1-antitrypsin inhibit the action of proteases released from bacteria and neutrophils which degrade proteins, and α_1-antitrypsin deficiency predisposes to disruption of elastin and development of emphysema (see Chapters 17 and 23). **Surfactant protein A**, apart from its actions on surface tension, enhances phagocytosis by coating or **opsonizing** (literally 'making ready to eat') bacteria and other particles. **Lysozyme** is secreted in large quantities in the airways and has antifungal and bactericidal properties; together with the antimicrobial proteins lactoferrin, peroxidases, and neutrophil-derived defensins, it provides non-specific immunity to the respiratory tract. **Secretory immunoglobulin A** (IgA) is the principal immunoglobulin in airway secretions and with IgM and IgG agglutinates and opsonizes antigenic particles; it also restricts adherence of microbes to the mucosa. Secretory IgA consists of a dimer of two IgA molecules produced by **plasma cells** (activated B-lymphocytes, see below) and a glycoprotein **secretory component**. The latter is produced on the basolateral surface of epithelial cells, where it binds the IgA dimer (see Fig. 17). The secretory IgA complex is then transferred to the luminal surface of the epithelial cell and released into the bronchial fluid (see Fig. 17). It can account for 10% of the total protein in bronchioalveolar lavage fluid.

Lung macrophages

Macrophages are mobile **mononuclear phagocytes** that are found throughout the respiratory tract. They act as sentinels in the airways, providing innate protection against inhaled microorganisms and other particles by **phagocytosis** (ingesting them) and production of potent antimicrobial agents including reactive oxygen species. Phagocytosed organic material is usually digested, whereas inorganic material is sequestered inside the cell. As alveolar epithelium does not have cilia, alveolar macrophages are key to removing material and are the major cell present in the alveoli. Other functions include clearance of surfactant proteins and suppression of unnecessary immune responses by production of **anti-inflammatory cytokines** such as interleukin-10 (IL-10) and transforming growth factor β (TGFβ). However, in more severe infections, they can initiate inflammatory responses and by release of chemoattractants such as leukotriene B_4 promote neutrophil infiltration from the plasma. They can also act as antigen-presenting cells (see below).

Development of immunity

T-lymphocytes and **B-lymphocytes** migrate to lymph nodes, tonsils and adenoids and diffuse patches of bronchus-associated lymphoid tissue (**BALT**) within the lamina propria. Here they interact and are programmed. Antigen is presented to **CD4+ T-lymphocytes** (T-helper or T_H cells) by **antigen-presenting cells**. The most important are **dendritic cells**, highly specialized mononuclear phagocytes (see Fig. 17). Macrophages, B-lymphocytes and some epithelial cells can also act as antigen-presenting cells. On presentation of antigen, T_H cells release **cytokines** such as IL-2, IL-4, IL-13 and interferon-γ (IFN-γ). IL-2 activates **CD8+ T-lymphocytes** (cytotoxic or T_C cells), which kill infected cells. IL-4, IL-13 and IFN-γ activate B-lymphocytes in the presence of antigen binding to surface immunoglobulins (IgM) (see Fig. 17). Activated B-lymphocytes proliferate and differentiate into **plasma cells** that re-enter the bloodstream. These secrete large amounts of antigen-specific antibody (immunoglobins). Binding of antibody to antigen may neutralize some toxic molecules, but more commonly activates secondary mechanisms, either directly by opsonization, allowing recognition and phago-cytosis by macrophages and neutrophils, or by activation of **complement**. When activated, complement can: kill pathogens by lysis (bursting the cell membrane); opsonize the antibody–antigen complex; and recruit inflammatory cells. For more detailed information on immunity, see *Immunology at a Glance*.

18 Pulmonary function tests

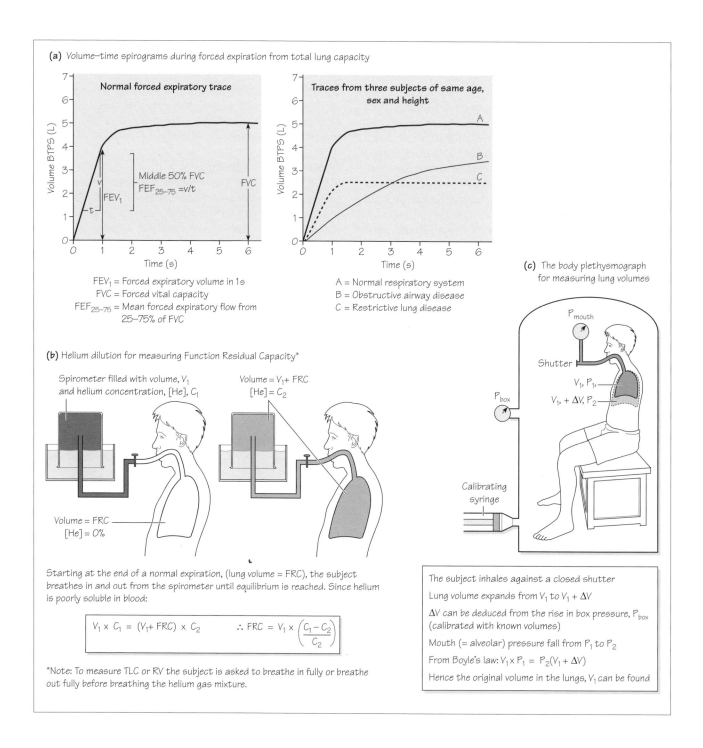

(a) Volume–time spirograms during forced expiration from total lung capacity

Normal forced expiratory trace

FEV₁ = Forced expiratory volume in 1s
FVC = Forced vital capacity
FEF₂₅₋₇₅ = Mean forced expiratory flow from 25–75% of FVC

Traces from three subjects of same age, sex and height

A = Normal respiratory system
B = Obstructive airway disease
C = Restrictive lung disease

(b) Helium dilution for measuring Function Residual Capacity*

Spirometer filled with volume, V_1 and helium concentration, [He], C_1

Volume = V_1 + FRC
[He] = C_2

Volume = FRC
[He] = 0%

Starting at the end of a normal expiration, (lung volume = FRC), the subject breathes in and out from the spirometer until equilibrium is reached. Since helium is poorly soluble in blood:

$$V_1 \times C_1 = (V_1 + FRC) \times C_2 \qquad \therefore FRC = V_1 \times \left(\frac{C_1 - C_2}{C_2}\right)$$

*Note: To measure TLC or RV the subject is asked to breathe in fully or breathe out fully before breathing the helium gas mixture.

(c) The body plethysmograph for measuring lung volumes

P_{mouth}
Shutter
V_1, P_1,
V_1, + ΔV, P_2
P_{box}
Calibrating syringe

The subject inhales against a closed shutter

Lung volume expands from V_1 to $V_1 + \Delta V$

ΔV can be deduced from the rise in box pressure, P_{box} (calibrated with known volumes)

Mouth (= alveolar) pressure fall from P_1 to P_2

From Boyle's law: $V_1 \times P_1 = P_2(V_1 + \Delta V)$

Hence the original volume in the lungs, V_1 can be found

Accurate assessment of defects in airflow, lung volume or gas exchange is essential to the diagnosis and management of many respiratory disorders. It is important to note that these tests characterize 'defects'; the clinician has to diagnose 'diseases'. The normal range of many lung function tests is very wide and it is essential to compare measured values with those predicted for the subject's age, height and sex by standard **nomograms** derived from large cross-sectional studies.

Airway resistance can be measured using a **body plethysmograph** (Chapter 7 and Fig. 18c) to measure alveolar pressure. **Lung compliance** can be measured using an **oesophageal balloon** to measure intrapleural pressure (for details, see Chapter 6). More commonly, abnormalities of airway resistance (in obstructive airway disease) are assessed indirectly from forced expiratory manoeuvres and abnormalities of compliance (in restrictive lung disease) are assessed indirectly from lung volume measurements.

Forced expiratory tests

Peak expiratory flow rate (PEFR) is frequently measured, despite its inability to distinguish between different types of ventilatory defect and its dependence on patient effort (Fig. 7c). It is reduced in obstructive disease, respiratory muscle weakness and often in restrictive lung disease (secondary to reduced volume). Its main value lies in monitoring diseases, especially asthma, once the diagnosis has been made.

In contrast, plots of **volume against time (spirogram)** or **airflow against volume** during a forced expiration can help to distinguish between different types of defects. The patient is asked to inhale to total lung capacity (TLC) and breathe out as hard and fast as possible to residual volume (RV). A plot of volume against time (Fig. 18a) can be produced by continuously measuring volume, either with a spirometer or by integrating a flowmeter output. If a flowmeter is used, it is also possible to compute a flow vs. volume plot from the same forced expiration (Fig. 7c). Flow–volume plots show characteristic shapes with different defects (see Fig. 7e), such as the 'scooped out' appearance seen in obstructive airway disease.

Forced vital capacity (FVC) and **forced expiratory volume in 't' seconds (FEV$_t$)** can be read off the volume vs. time plot (Fig. 18a). FEV$_1$ is extremely reproducible and correlates well with function and prognosis. It is normal for FVC and FEV$_1$ to peak in adults in the third decade and then decline by approximately 30 mL/year (Fig. 23b). FEV$_1$/FVC is normally 0.75–0.90, but higher values may occur in normal children. FEV$_1$/FVC helps distinguish between obstructive and restrictive ventilatory defects. Typically, in obstructive lung diseases (e.g. COPD, acute asthma) the FEV$_1$/FVC is less than 0.70. If the airway obstruction is due to asthma, FEV$_1$, FVC and FEV$_1$/FVC may all increase after the inhalation of bronchodilators. In restrictive lung disease (e.g. lung fibrosis), absolute values of FEV$_1$ and FVC are reduced, but FEV$_1$/FVC is normal or high.

Forced mid-expiratory flow (FEF$_{25-75}$) is the average forced expiratory flow rate over the middle 50% of the FVC. It may be especially affected by small airway disease, but the normal range is wide.

Maximal voluntary ventilation (MVV) is measured by asking the subject to breathe as hard and fast as possible into a spirometer for 15 s, with the ventilation expressed in L/min. It is very dependent on effort and not very reproducible, but it may correlate well with subjective dyspnoea.

Lung volumes

Restrictive ventilatory defects (RVDs) are characterized by a reduction in TLC. Lung volumes such as TLC, RV and FRC can be measured by **helium dilution** (Fig. 18b) or by **body plethysmography** (Fig. 18c). The gas dilution method is simpler for patients, but it is sensitive to gas leaks and will underestimate TLC in the presence of extensive bullous or cystic lung disease. RVDs may be caused by parenchymal lung disease (pulmonary fibrosis, scleroderma, pulmonary oedema), chest wall disease (kyphoscoliosis, massive obesity) or weak respiratory muscles (myasthenia gravis, muscular dystrophy). RV and FRC can help distinguish between these conditions, as FRC and RV are usually reduced in lung disease; whereas FRC is usually normal and RV elevated in muscle weakness. FVC and TLC usually decline in parallel, therefore once an RVD has been established by measurement of TLC, the progress of the disease may be followed with FVC from spirometry.

Measurement of lung compliance (Chapter 6) and **transdiaphragmatic pressure** (P_{di}) may distinguish further between RVD due to parenchymal lung disease or muscle weakness. By using two small balloon-tipped catheters, one measuring oesophageal ($P_{pleural}$) pressure and the other gastric (P_{abd}) pressure, P_{di} (= $P_{abd}-P_{pleural}$) can be measured during a maximal inspiration or sniff from FRC. Typically, in parenchymal lung disease lung compliance is low, elastic recoil pressure high and P_{di} normal; whereas in respiratory muscle weakness lung compliance is relatively normal, elastic recoil pressure low, and P_{di} low.

Diffusing capacity is a measure of the ability of gas to diffuse from the alveolus into pulmonary capillary blood. As discussed in Chapter 5, $D_L co$ is used as a surrogate for $D_L o_2$, since it is simple to measure and carbon monoxide diffuses across the lung in a fashion similar to oxygen. It often helps interpretation to normalize $D_L co$ to the alveolar volume (V_A) by calculating the coefficient, $K co = D_L co/V_A$. $D_L co$ is reduced by reduced alveolar surface area, thickened alveolar–capillary membrane, reduced capillary blood volume or anaemia. Reductions in the $D_L co$ can be caused by a variety of parenchymal diseases (idiopathic pulmonary fibrosis, emphysema, pneumonia) or vascular diseases (pulmonary hypertension, pulmonary oedema), such that the test is sensitive but not specific. Reductions in the $D_L co$ below 50% predicted for age, sex and height are often associated with oxygen desaturation during exercise. Severe reductions in $D_L co$ (<20% predicted) may result in resting hypoxaemia.

19 Chest imaging and bronchoscopy

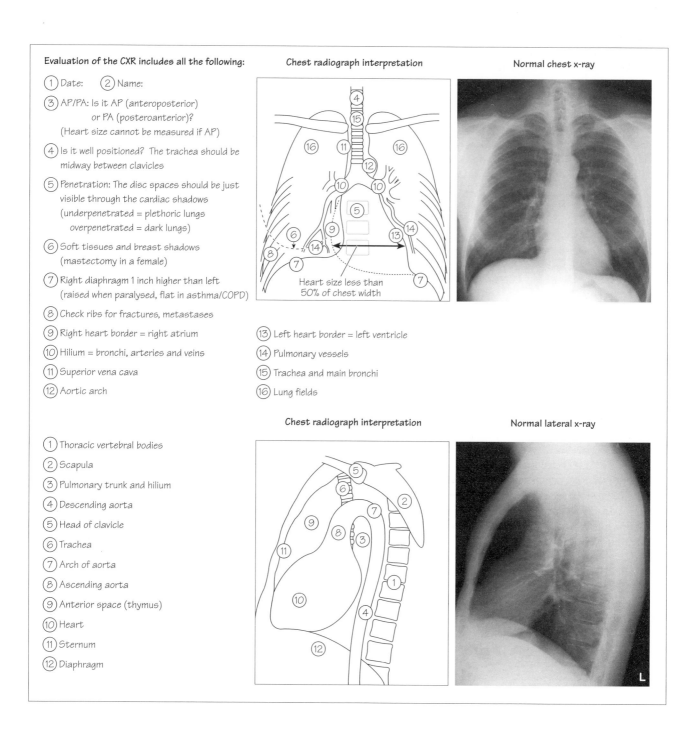

Evaluation of the CXR includes all the following:

1. Date: 2. Name:

3. AP/PA: Is it AP (anteroposterior) or PA (posteroanterior)? (Heart size cannot be measured if AP)

4. Is it well positioned? The trachea should be midway between clavicles

5. Penetration: The disc spaces should be just visible through the cardiac shadows (underpenetrated = plethoric lungs overpenetrated = dark lungs)

6. Soft tissues and breast shadows (mastectomy in a female)

7. Right diaphragm 1 inch higher than left (raised when paralysed, flat in asthma/COPD)

8. Check ribs for fractures, metastases

9. Right heart border = right atrium

10. Hilium = bronchi, arteries and veins

11. Superior vena cava

12. Aortic arch

13. Left heart border = left ventricle

14. Pulmonary vessels

15. Trachea and main bronchi

16. Lung fields

Chest radiograph interpretation

Heart size less than 50% of chest width

Normal chest x-ray

1. Thoracic vertebral bodies
2. Scapula
3. Pulmonary trunk and hilium
4. Descending aorta
5. Head of clavicle
6. Trachea
7. Arch of aorta
8. Ascending aorta
9. Anterior space (thymus)
10. Heart
11. Sternum
12. Diaphragm

Chest radiograph interpretation

Normal lateral x-ray

Radiography of the chest was one of the first medical utilizations of X-ray imaging and it is still used daily to detect, diagnose or follow morphologic abnormalities in the chest. Standard two-dimensional chest X-rays are still the mainstay of chest radiographic procedures. Recent innovations have included digital imaging, three-dimensional imaging (computed tomography scans) and physiologic images (positron emission tomography and ventilation–perfusion scans). Specific radiographic abnormalities are discussed in later chapters.

Posteroanterior (PA) and lateral chest radiographs (CXRs) allow two-dimensional visualization of the lungs, great vessels, heart, diaphragm and mediastinum. PA films should be performed upright at total lung capacity. Features seen in CXR and basic CXR interpretation are shown in the Fig. 19. In patients under 40 years of age with no suspected lung disease, lateral films need not be performed for screening purposes. Portable films shot anterior–posterior (AP) in patients unable to stand magnify the heart and mediastinum and do not allow detailed visualization of lung parenchyma.

A standard PA and lateral CXR should allow visualization of both lungs, including the diaphragmatic position, as well as the normal trachea, main carina, mainstem bronchi, major and minor fissures, aorta, main pulmonary arteries and heart. Understanding of the normal anatomy of a CXR is essential to allow recognition of abnormal lung parenchymal infiltrates, enlarged lymph nodes adjacent to the trachea or in the hila, enlarged pulmonary arteries, volume loss of a lobe or segment or cardiac enlargement. In the case of a suspected pleural effusion, lateral decubitus films allow visualization of as little as 50 mL of free-flowing fluid. Digital CXRs are being developed that allow more detailed views of the denser portions of the thorax and show finer detail of the lung parenchyma.

Computed tomography (CT): a limitation of standard CXR imaging is that the two-dimensional image obscures details and averages densities in the third dimension (anterior–posterior on the PA film). CT allows thin slice axial images and fine-detailed examination of intrathoracic structures. Administration of intravenous contrast allows imaging of the pulmonary blood vessels (such as in suspected pulmonary embolus) and demonstration of abnormal lymph nodes (such as in evaluation of malignancy or infection). CT also permits resolution of interstitial lung infiltrates as well as precise localization of infiltrates, masses, cavities, bulla, fluid collections and airway abnormalities. Examples of CT scans are shown in several chapters. Newer technology allows complete axial scanning of the thorax with a single breath-hold.

Ventilation–perfusion (V/Q) scans are mostly performed in the evaluation of pulmonary embolism (PE) (Fig. 25). Gamma cameras can visualize radiopharmaceuticals either injected into the venous blood (perfusion) or inhaled (ventilation). Thromboembolism classically causes a V/Q mismatch, with absence of perfusion in the presence of ventilation. Unfortunately, the value of V/Q scans is limited by the observation that many PEs result in indeterminate V/Q scans that show small mismatches or matched V/Q deficits. In these cases, other studies must be utilized to demonstrate thromboemboli. Contrast CT scans are increasingly used as screening tools for PE and are being investigated as possible replacements for V/Q scanning. Quantitative V/Q scans may be used in preparation for lung resection surgery, to assess regional lung function and estimate the amount of residual lung function.

Pulmonary angiography, where the vasculature is visualized following injection of contrast medium (see Chapter 25), may be required in some patients with suspected pulmonary emboli but equivocal V/Q scans, pulmonary hypertension and pulmonary vascular disease, including vasculitis and arteriovenous malformations. These studies are often preceded by echocardiography to visualize right ventricular function and estimate pulmonary artery pressure using Doppler imaging.

Positron emission tomography (PET) utilizing a fluorinated analogue of glucose (FDG) gives images of the lung that highlight areas of increased glucose metabolism. Malignant cells have increased glucose uptake and appear as increased densities on PET images. Recent studies have demonstrated that FDG PET is useful in distinguishing between benign and malignant solitary pu monary nodules and in detecting small nodal metastases that may not be apparent on CT scanning. For these indications, PET has a sensitivity and specificity from 80 to 97% with false positive scans seen in cases of infection or granulomatous inflammation. Whole body FDG PET was recently used to detect clinically inapparent distant metastases.

Bronchoscopy enables direct visualization of the endobronchial tree. Chest physicians perform most bronchoscopies, as day cases under local anaesthetic in the sedated but awake patient, using a flexible fibre-optic instrument. It has the advantages of visualization of the upper lobes and is a safe technique with a low complication rate. Saturation and heart rhythm should be monitored and supplemental oxygen administered during the procedure. Facilities for resuscitation should always be immediately available. Thoracic surgeons may use a rigid bronchoscope in the fully anaesthetized patient. This instrument allows larger biopsies and better suctioning, and is the method of choice when removing inhaled foreign bodies. Bronchoscopy is most frequently performed to investigate if a shadow on a chest radiograph is due to a lung cancer (Chapter 36). If an endobronchial tumour is seen, biopsies for histological analysis and washings and brush samples for cytological analysis can be taken. In addition, information regarding the operability of the tumour can be obtained. Bronchoscopy can also be used to diagnose parenchymal lung disease using the technique of transbronchial biopsy, which obtains parenchymal and bronchial tissue for histological examination. Collection of bronchoalveolar fluid (BAL, bronchoalveolar lavage) is useful in diagnosing alveolitis (raised lymphocyte count in sarcoidosis), infection in the immunocompromised patient (e.g. *Pneumocystis carinii* pneumonia) and tuberculosis. Bronchoscopy also aids investigation of collapsed segments or lobes. Therapeutically, bronchoscopy is used to remove inhaled foreign bodies, to aspirate sputum plugs and secretions, to relieve stenosis by placement of stents and during treatment of endobronchial tumours with laser or endobronchial radiotherapy. Haemorrhage, pneumothorax and cardiac arrhythmia, although uncommon, are the main complications of fibre-optic bronchoscopy.

20 Respiratory failure

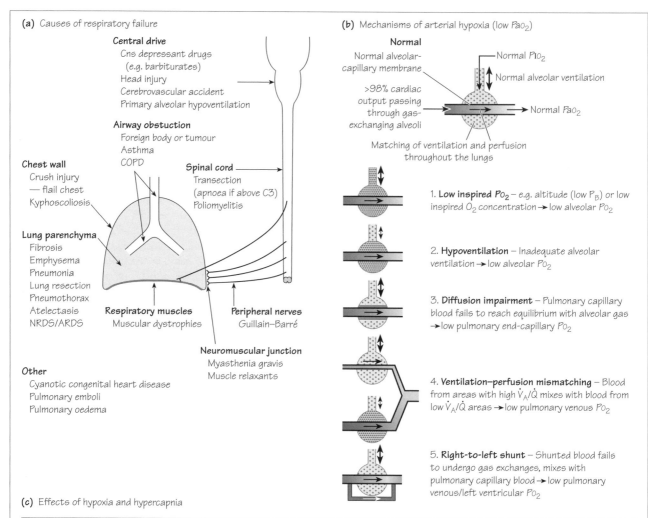

(a) Causes of respiratory failure

Central drive
Cns depressant drugs
(e.g. barbiturates)
Head injury
Cerebrovascular accident
Primary alveolar hypoventilation

Airway obstuction
Foreign body or tumour
Asthma
COPD

Spinal cord
Transection
(apnoea if above C3)
Poliomyelitis

Chest wall
Crush injury
— flail chest
Kyphoscoliosis

Lung parenchyma
Fibrosis
Emphysema
Pneumonia
Lung resection
Pneumothorax
Atelectasis
NRDS/ARDS

Respiratory muscles
Muscular dystrophies

Peripheral nerves
Guillain–Barré

Neuromuscular junction
Myasthenia gravis
Muscle relaxants

Other
Cyanotic congenital heart disease
Pulmonary emboli
Pulmonary oedema

(b) Mechanisms of arterial hypoxia (low Pao_2)

Normal
Normal alveolar-capillary membrane
>98% cardiac output passing through gas-exchanging alveoli
Normal Pio_2
Normal alveolar ventilation
Normal Pao_2
Matching of ventilation and perfusion throughout the lungs

1. **Low inspired Po_2** – e.g. altitude (low P_B) or low inspired O_2 concentration → low alveolar Po_2

2. **Hypoventilation** – Inadequate alveolar ventilation → low alveolar Po_2

3. **Diffusion impairment** – Pulmonary capillary blood fails to reach equilibrium with alveolar gas → low pulmonary end-capillary Po_2

4. **Ventilation–perfusion mismatching** – Blood from areas with high $\dot{V}_A/\dot{Q}$ mixes with blood from low $\dot{V}_A/\dot{Q}$ areas → low pulmonary venous Po_2

5. **Right-to-left shunt** – Shunted blood fails to undergo gas exchanges, mixes with pulmonary capillary blood → low pulmonary venous/left ventricular Po_2

(c) Effects of hypoxia and hypercapnia

	Acute	Chronic—compensation and complications
Low Pao_2 (hypoxaemia/ hypoxia)	**Impaired CNS function:** irritability, confusion, drowsiness, convulsions, coma, death **Central cyanosis** (not very sensitive; may be absent in anaemia) **Cardiac arrhythmias** **Hypoxic vasoconstriction*** of pulmonary vessels	**Erythropoietin** from hypoxic kidney → **polycythaemia** → ↑ oxygen carriage despite low Pao_2 but if excessive (haematocrit >55%) the ↑viscosity impairs tissue blood flow **Polycythaemia** → florid complexion; increased cyanosis ***Pulmonary hypertension** → right ventricular hypertrophy **Fluid retention/right heart failure (cor pulmonale*)** → peripheral oedema/ascites/ ↑jugular venous pressure/enlarged liver
High $Paco_2$ (hypercapnia)	**Low arterial pH** (respiratory acidosis) **Peripheral vasodilatation** → warm flushed skin, bounding pulse **Cerebral vasodilatation** → ↑ intra-cranial pressure → headache, worse on waking if nocturnal ventilation↓ **Impaired CNS/muscle function:** irritability, confusion, somnolence, coma, tremor, myolonic jerks, hand flap **Cardiac arrythmias**	**Renal compensation** (compensatory metabolic alkalosis) → ↑arterial $[HCO_3^-]$ → arterial pH returned to near normal **Cerebrospinal fluid (CSF) compensation** → ↑CSF $[HCO_3^-]$ → CSF pH returned to near normal → respiratory drive less at any given $Paco_2$ than in acute hypercapnia *Hypercapnia accentuates the effects of hypoxia on pulmonary blood vessels and therefore contributes to the development of cor pulmonale (see above)

Respiratory failure is usually said to exist when arterial P_{O_2} falls below 8 kPa (60 mmHg) when breathing air at sea level. In **type 1 respiratory failure**, the arterial hypoxia is accompanied by a normal or low arterial P_{CO_2}, whereas in **type 2 or ventilatory failure**, arterial P_{CO_2} is increased above 6.7 kPa (50 mmHg). Respiratory failure may be **acute** or **chronic**. In chronic respiratory failure, there are permanent abnormalities in blood gases, which typically worsen periodically (**acute on chronic**). This strict definition excludes some patients whose respiratory systems might otherwise be considered failing. Some patients have disabling **dyspnoea** (breathlessness) of respiratory origin but maintain $P_{O_2} > 8$ kPa.

Some of the many causes of respiratory failure are listed in Fig. 20a. Symptoms and signs clearly depend on the underlying cause. Dyspnoea and **tachypnoea** (increased respiratory rate) will be prominent in severe asthma but absent in conditions with reduced central drive.

Mechanisms leading to hypoxia and hypercapnia

Of the five causes of hypoxaemia (Fig. 20b), only **hypoventilation** inevitably causes increased $P_{a}CO_2$.

$$P_{a}CO_2 \propto \frac{\dot{V}_{CO_2}}{\dot{V}_A} \text{ (Chapter 9)}$$

If hypoxia is out of proportion to the hypercapnia and the **A–a P_{O_2} gradient** (see Chapter 14) is increased, one of the other mechanisms (see 3–5 in Fig. 20b) must also be present. The primary effect of **right-to-left shunts** and **ventilation–perfusion mismatching** is to raise arterial CO_2 content, but this is usually corrected or over-corrected by a reflex increase in ventilation (Chapters 13 and 14).

Thickening of the alveolar–capillary membrane in lung fibrosis may give rise to **diffusion impairment**, preventing equilibration of pulmonary capillary blood with alveolar gas, especially in exercise, when time in the capillary is reduced. However, in many conditions thought to cause diffusion impairment, there is also substantial V_A/Q mismatching, and this is probably the main cause of the hypoxia.

Effects of hypoxia and hypercapnia

The direct effects of hypoxia and hypercapnia, together with the compensations and complications that occur in chronic respiratory failure, are shown in Fig. 20c.

Although hypoxia usually offers the greatest threat to vital organs, hypercapnia and especially acidosis are also important and they often accentuate the adverse effects of each other. Hypoxia and hypercapnia are better tolerated when they develop slowly in chronic respiratory failure because of adaptations such as polycythaemia and compensatory metabolic alkalosis.

Cyanosis is a greyish-blue tinge seen when a tissue's microcirculation contains a high concentration of deoxygenated haemoglobin. It may occur with impaired blood flow, for example in the hands and feet in circulatory shock, when it is known as **peripheral cyanosis**. When the arterial blood contains more than about 1.5–2 g/dL of deoxygenated haemoglobin, the concentration in the microcirculation reaches the critical level for cyanosis to be observable even in well-perfused tissues. This occurs with an arterial saturation of about 85% if haemoglobin concentration is normal (15 g/dL) and the resulting **central cyanosis** is visible in the tongue and mucus membranes of the mouth. It appears at higher oxygen saturations in polycythaemic patients, whereas in severe anaemia central cyanosis may be impossible, as it would require an O_2 saturation incompatible with life.

Respiratory failure in asthma

Hypoxia in a severe asthma attack is primarily due to V_A/Q mismatching. $P_{a}CO_2$ usually falls as the attack worsens, because peripheral chemoreceptor and pulmonary receptor stimulation produce a reflex increase in ventilation despite the increased work of breathing. A raised or even apparently normal $P_{a}CO_2$ (e.g. 5.3 kPa, 40 mmHg) in a severe hypoxic asthma attack is a cause for concern, as it may indicate the onset of exhaustion and potentially life-threatening asthma.

Respiratory failure in chronic obstructive pulmonary disease

The clinical picture of severe chronic obstructive pulmonary disease (COPD) is variable, but two extreme patterns—the **pink puffer** and the **blue bloater**—are recognized and described in Chapter 23. The blue bloater is associated with type 2 respiratory failure. He has a chronically low $P_{a}O_2$ and high $P_{a}CO_2$ and these worsen with acute infections, which precipitate acute on chronic respiratory failure. Patients with chronic hypercapnia typically have a near-normal arterial pH owing to an efficient compensatory metabolic alkalosis via renal generation and retention of bicarbonate. During an acute exacerbation, $P_{a}CO_2$ may increase further and pH then falls significantly, as renal adjustments are slow. Arterial pH can therefore indicate the proportions of acute and chronic hypercapnia. Patients with chronic hypercapnia are at risk of respiratory depression and a further, potentially fatal, increase in $P_{a}CO_2$ if given high inspired oxygen (Chapter 39). This may be due to loss of hypoxic drive in the presence of reduced CO_2 sensitivity, but other mechanisms may contribute, including increased V_A/Q mismatching by the removal of hypoxic vasoconstriction. As these patients are on the steep part of the oxyhaemoglobin dissociation curve, significant improvements in arterial oxygen content can usually be achieved by small increases in $F_I O_2$ (to 24 or 28%). The resulting small improvement in $P_{a}O_2$ does not cause respiratory depression (see Chapter 12).

Management

All patients suspected of having respiratory failure will need arterial blood gas measurement, as the severity is difficult to assess clinically. A chest X-ray helps detect possible causes and aggravating factors such as pneumonia or pneumothorax. Other investigations, including lung function tests, will depend on the clinical situation and likely underlying disease. Management will include airway maintenance, clearance of secretions, oxygen therapy (Chapter 39) and in some cases mechanical ventilation (Chapter 38). Specific therapies, such as bronchodilators and antibiotics, are directed at the underlying cause or aggravating factors. Abnormalities in haemoglobin concentration, fluid balance and cardiac output should be treated to improve tissue oxygen delivery and increase mixed venous oxygen content, which in turn will also reduce the effects of venous admixture on arterial oxygenation.

21 Asthma: pathophysiology

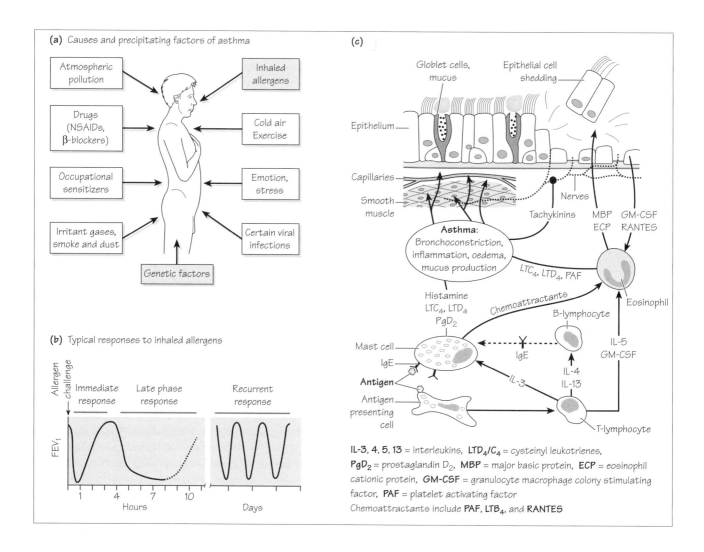

(a) Causes and precipitating factors of asthma

- Atmospheric pollution
- Inhaled allergens
- Drugs (NSAIDs, β-blockers)
- Cold air Exercise
- Occupational sensitizers
- Emotion, stress
- Irritant gases, smoke and dust
- Certain viral infections
- Genetic factors

(b) Typical responses to inhaled allergens

Allergen challenge
FEV$_1$
Immediate response | Late phase response | Recurrent response
Hours 1 4 7 10
Days

(c)

Globlet cells, mucus — Epithelial cell shedding — Epithelium — Capillaries — Smooth muscle

Asthma: Bronchoconstriction, inflammation, oedema, mucus production

Tachykinins — MBP ECP — GM-CSF RANTES — Nerves — Eosinophil

Histamine LTC$_4$, LTD$_4$ PgD$_2$ — LTC$_4$, LTD$_4$, PAF — Chemoattractants — B-lymphocyte — IL-5 GM-CSF

Mast cell — IgE — IgE — IL-4 IL-13 — IL-3

Antigen — Antigen presenting cell — T-lymphocyte

IL-3, 4, 5, 13 = interleukins, LTD$_4$/C$_4$ = cysteinyl leukotrienes, PgD$_2$ = prostaglandin D$_2$, MBP = major basic protein, ECP = eosinophil cationic protein, GM-CSF = granulocyte macrophage colony stimulating factor, PAF = platelet activating factor
Chemoattractants include PAF, LTB$_4$, and RANTES

Asthma is an inflammatory disease of the airways. Patients suffer from episodes of cough, wheezing, chest tightness and/or dyspnoea (breathlessness), which are often worse at night or early in the morning. There is considerable variation in the severity and frequency of attacks. Asthma can be usefully defined as 'increased responsiveness of the bronchi to various stimuli, manifested by widespread narrowing of the airways that changes in severity either spontaneously or as a result of treatment'.

The major characteristics of asthma are:

1 Narrowing of the airways and impeded air flow, commonly reversible spontaneously or following treatment.

2 Increased sensitivity to bronchoconstricting stimuli (**hyperresponsiveness**).

3 Increased numbers of **inflammatory cells** (eosinophils, mast cells, neutrophils, T lymphocytes) in the bronchi.

There is also **hypersecretion of mucus**, blockage of airways with **mucus plugs** and swelling of mucosa due to inflammation-associated vascular leak and **oedema**, all of which further limit air

flow. Damage to the epithelium (**epithelial shedding**) is reflected by whorls of epithelial cells (Curschmann's spirals) in the mucus, which also contains eosinophil cell membranes (Charcot–Leyden crystals). In chronic severe asthma, **remodelling of the airways** occurs, including increased bronchial smooth muscle content. This causes irreversible narrowing of the airways and limits the effectiveness of bronchodilators.

Prevalence

Asthma is increasing in prevalence, particularly in the Western world, where >5% of the population may be symptomatic and receiving treatment. There has been a concomitant increase in mortality, despite improved treatment. In the UK, one in seven of the population has allergic disease and over 9 million people will have wheezed in the last year. The number of teenagers with asthma has nearly doubled over the last 12 years. Prevalence of asthma varies greatly geographically, being least common in the Far East and most common in the UK, Australia and New Zealand. There is some correlation with Westernized life-styles, including living conditions that favour house-dust mites and atmospheric pollution.

Classification

Asthma can be classified as **extrinsic**, having a definite external cause and **intrinsic**, where no external cause can be identified. Extrinsic asthma most commonly occurs as a result of an allergic response, with development of **IgE antibodies** to specific antigens (**allergic** or **atopic asthma**) and tends to start in childhood with symptoms becoming less severe with age. Intrinsic asthma generally appears in adults and does not improve.

Atopic asthma

Individuals who readily produce IgE to common antigens are prone to allergic asthma. Major antigens include fecal pellets from **house-dust mite**—the most common cause of asthma worldwide, grass pollen and dander from **domestic pets**. Genetic factors, atmospheric pollution and maternal smoking in pregnancy all predispose to raised IgE levels and later development of asthma and airway hyperresponsiveness (Fig. 21a).

Inhalation of allergens by atopic individuals initiates an **immediate response** (bronchoconstriction) that usually subsides within 2 h (Fig. 21b); this is reversible with bronchodilators such as the β_2-adrenoceptor antagonist salbutamol (Chapter 22). This is often followed 3–12 h later by a **late-phase response**, including bronchoconstriction and development of airway inflammation and hyperresponsiveness, which is less susceptible to bronchodilators. Some materials such as isocyanates cause only an **isolated late phase**. The increase in airway hyperresponsiveness associated with the late phase may promote **recurrent asthma attacks** over several days.

The immediate response is caused by antigen/IgE-induced **mast cell degranulation** and release of **histamine, prostaglandin D$_2$** (PgD$_2$) and **leukotriene C$_4$ and D$_4$** (LTC$_4$, LTD$_4$); these cause bronchoconstriction, increased mucus production and vascular leak (Fig. 21c). In the late phase, mediators from mast cells and activated **T lymphocytes** cause infiltration of **neutrophils** and **eosinophils**. Eosinophils are present in large numbers in asthmatic bronchi and release **leukotrienes**, platelet-activating factor (**PAF**), **major basic protein** (**MBP**) and **eosinophil cationic protein** (**ECP**). MBP and ECP contribute to epithelial cell damage, with consequent increased permeability to allergens, release of eosinophil chemoattractants (e.g. RANTES) and cytokines such as granulocyte macrophage colony-stimulating factor (GM-CSF) and exposure of C-fibre afferent nerve endings. The latter release proinflammatory tachykinins.

Occupational asthma

Many materials may give rise to occupational asthma. Some are allergens (e.g. flour, grain, animals, certain commercial enzymes), whereas others are not, including **isocyanates** (present in industrial and polyurethane coatings) and fumes from welding or soldering. Twenty per cent of the working population may be susceptible to occupational asthma.

Drug-associated asthma

Aspirin and other non-steroidal anti-inflammatory drugs (NSAIDs) promote asthmatic attacks in 5% of asthmatics. They inhibit the cyclooxygenase (COX) pathway that synthesizes prostaglandins and shift arachidonic acid metabolism from COX towards the lipoxygenase pathway and production of LTC$_4$ and LTD$_4$. Aspirin-induced asthma is reversed by antileukotriene therapy (Chapter 22).

The bronchi are innervated by parasympathetic nerves that release acetylcholine, which causes bronchoconstriction and stimulates mucus production and non-adrenergic, non-cholinergic (NANC) nerves. Parasympathetic activity may increase in asthma due to axon reflexes from irritant receptors in the bronchi (Chapter 11). There is little sympathetic innervation, although circulating epinephrine (adrenaline) acting via β_2-adrenoceptors on smooth muscle causes bronchodilation. Consequently β-adrenoceptor antagonists such as propranolol can cause bronchoconstriction in asthmatics. This may even occur with nominally β_1-selective drugs and treatment of cardiovascular disease with such agents should be avoided in asthmatics.

Other factors

Asthmatics have hyperresponsive airways and irritant gases and dusts that do not affect healthy individuals can precipitate asthmatic attacks or worsen symptoms. Such factors include **tobacco smoke, exhaust fumes** and pollutants such as **nitrogen dioxide, sulphur dioxide** and **ozone**. Exercise and inhalation of cold air often precipitate wheezing in asthmatics, probably via drying and cooling of the bronchial epithelium. This is common in children. Emotional stress can also induce an asthmatic attack. Certain **viral infections** (rhinovirus, parainfluenza, respiratory syncytial virus) are also associated with asthma attacks. The **pathogenesis** of asthma is complex; Fig. 21c shows only a simplified scenario.

22 Asthma: treatment

(a) Step-wise approach to asthma therapy

Step up: If control is not maintained, consider stepping up therapy, but review avoidance of allergens and patient compliance

Step	Symptoms	Typical PEFR (% predicted)	Long-term control	Quick relief
1	Less frequent than daily	100%	None required	For all stages: Short-acting broncho-dilator as required (inhaled β_2 agonist) Used more than once daily or increasing use indicates need for additional long-term therapy
2	Daily	≤80%	Anti-inflammatory drugs: Low-dose inhaled steroids (<800 µg daily) Other controller drugs if steroids cannot be used	
3	Moderate to severe	50–80%	Add long-acting β_2-agonists (salmeterol)	
4	Severe	50–80%	Add any or all of: (empirical trial) increased inhaled steroids to <2000 µg daily, oral β_2-agonists, theophylline, leukotriene receptor antagonists	
5	Severe deteriorating	≤50%	Add oral prednisolone (40 mg daily)	
6	Further deterioration	≤30%	Hospitalization	

Based on British Thoracic Society Guidelines, Thorax 2002

Step down: Review treatment regime every 1–6 months; a gradual stepwise reduction in therapy may be possible

(b) Drugs used in asthma therapy

Type	β_2-adrenoreceptor agonists	Muscarinic receptor antagonists	Xanthines	Corticocosteroids	Cromones	Anti-leukotrienes
	Inhaled, oral and IV: **Short acting:** Salbutamol (albuterol) Terbutaline, Rimeterol, Fenoterol, Pirbuterol **Long acting:** Salmeterol, Formoterol	*Inhaled:* Ipratropium bromide Oxitropium bromide	*Oral and IV:* Theophylline Aminophylline Enprofylline Slow release preparations	*Inhaled:* Beclomethasone proprionate, Fluticasone proprionate, Budesonide *Oral:* Prednisone, Prednisolone *Intravenous:* Hydrocortisone Methylprednisolone	*Inhaled:* Sodium cromoglycate (cromolyn) Nedocromil sodium	*Oral:* **Receptor antagonists:** Montelukast, Pranlukast, Zafirlukast **Lipoxygenase inhibitors:** Zileuton
Adverse affects (dose related)	Muscle tremor (most common) Tachycardia, palpitations (less common) Hypokalaemia (?, high infused does)	Rare Ipratropium – bitter taste	Headaches, nausea, vomiting, abdominal discomfort, diuresis, cardiac arrhythmias, epilepsy, behavioural disturbance (?) Interactions with many drugs affect plasma levels; important due to narrow therapeutic range	*Inhaled:* Oral candidiasis, hoarseness, cough *Oral and high dose:* Growth retardation, bruising, suppression of hypothalamic-pituitary axis, ostoeporosis, water retention, hypertension, weight gain, eye problems, diabetes, psychosis	Rare Throat irritation with inhaled powder	None significant described so far, though zafirlukast has benn asscciated with some cases of Churg-Strauss syndrome, a very rare vasculitis. These cases may however be related to a reduced steroid dose rather than the drug dose itself

(c) Pressurized metered dose inhaler

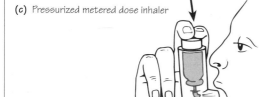

- Remove the cap and shake the inhaler
- Tilt the head back slightly and exhale
- Position the inhaler in the mouth (or preferably just in front of the open mouth)
- During a slow inspiration, press down the inhaler to release the medication
- Continue inhalation to full inspiration
- Hold breath for 10 seconds
- Actuate only one puff per inhalation

Management of asthma should encompass: assessment of severity and efficacy of therapy; identification and removal of precipitating factors; therapy to reverse bronchoconstriction and inflammation; patient and family participation and education.

Assessment

Lung function: Asthma is diagnosed when inhaled bronchodilators cause >15% improvement in forced expiratory volume in 1 s (FEV_1) or peak expiratory flow rate (PEFR) (Chapter 18). The absence of improvement does not rule out asthma—the disease could be in remission and chronic severe asthma is poorly reversible. Airway resistance has a circadian rhythm, being least at midday and greatest at 3–4 a.m. Serial measurements of PEFR in the morning, midday and on retiring are useful for identifying the enhanced variation in airflow limitation characteristic of asthma and for assessing response to therapy over time. Poorly controlled asthma shows a characteristic morning fall in PEFR ('morning dipping'). Occupational asthma is suggested when PEFR improves after a break from work. Lung function tests are often coupled with exercise tests in children, who often exhibit exercise-induced asthma.

Bronchial provocation tests are used to determine hyperresponsiveness when asthma is suspected but PEFR measurements are not diagnostic. Patients inhale increasing doses of histamine or methacholine (acetylcholine analogue) until FEV_1 declines by 20%. The dose at which this occurs ($PD_{20}FEV_1$) is greatly reduced in asthmatics, who are always hyperresponsive.

Skin prick tests are essential for identifying extrinsic factors. Development of a wheal around the prick site indicates allergen sensitivity. Exposure to identified allergens should be immediately minimized (e.g. replacement of furnishings to reduce house-dust mite; removal of pets), as once extrinsic asthma is established it may not be reversible. Only 50% of patients with occupational asthma are cured by avoidance of the precipitating factor.

Therapy

The goal is long-term control and all patients except those with the mildest symptoms should receive anti-inflammatory drugs as well as bronchodilators. International guidelines favour **step-wise treatment regimens** (Fig. 22a). Asthma therapy is centred on **inhaled** compounds (Fig. 22b). Inhalation maximizes bronchial delivery whilst minimizing systemic side effects. Metered dose inhalers are the most commonly used delivery systems, although only ~15% of the dose may reach the lungs (Fig. 22c).

β_2-Adrenoceptor agonists such as salbutamol are rapid and powerful bronchodilators and are of first choice for alleviating acute symptoms. They activate adenylate cyclase to increase cyclic adenosine monophosphate (cAMP) and may also reduce mediator release from inflammatory cells and airway nerves. Long-acting β_2-agonists such as salmeterol allow twice-daily dosage regimens. Long-term use of β_2-agonists is associated with reduced effectiveness (**tolerance**).

Muscarinic receptor antagonists such as ipratropium prevent acetylcholine released by parasympathetic nerves from causing bronchoconstriction and hypersecretion of mucus. They are less effective than β_2-agonists but longer-lasting and more effective against irritants than allergens. May be additive to β_2-agonists.

Corticosteroids such as beclomethasone are the most important anti-inflammatory drugs. They reduce eosinophil numbers and activation and activity of macrophages and lymphocytes. **Inhaled cor-** ticosteroids are the mainstay of long-term asthma therapy. They can, however, have significant side effects, including oral candidiasis (5%) and hoarseness. Growth may be retarded in children receiving high-dose inhaled corticosteroids. **Oral corticosteroids** such as prednisolone may be required in patients whose asthma cannot be controlled by inhaled steroids. The danger of adverse effects is much greater and excess corticosteroids may permanently suppress the hypothalamic–pituitary axis. **Combination therapies** containing both steroid plus long-acting β_2-agonists are useful for moderate/severe asthmatics.

Cromoglycate and **nedocromil** inhibit release of inflammatory mediators and prevent activation of mast cells and eosinophils. They may also suppress sensory nerve activity and release of neuropeptides (Chapter 21). Prophylactic use reduces both immediate and late phases of the asthmatic response and hyperresponsiveness. They are less powerful than steroids and only effective in mild and exercise-induced asthma. However, they have few side effects and are often the drug of choice for children. Use has declined since the introduction of safer, low-dose steroids, which are cheaper, more effective and do not need to be taken so often.

Xanthines such as theophylline have bronchodilatory and some anti-inflammatory actions and are taken orally. They inhibit phosphodiesterases that break down cAMP. Limitations include numerous side effects and a narrow therapeutic range; these are partially overcome by slow-release preparations. Xanthines are used as second-line drugs in asthma, particularly where β_2-agonists are ineffective at controlling symptoms and in steroid-resistant asthma.

Antileukotriene therapy has not been fully characterized and comes in two forms: cysLT receptor (LTC_4/D_4) antagonists such as montelukast, and 5-lipoxygenase inhibitors such as zileuton. Both have equal efficacy for bronchoconstriction caused by allergens, exercise and cold air, with ~50% reversal. They are also effective in aspirin-sensitive asthma, indicating the key role leukotrienes have in this condition (Chapter 21). Antileukotrienes improve lung function in mild and moderate asthmatics, but the greatest benefit may be for very severe asthmatics taking steroids. Both drug types are taken orally and are relatively long-lasting, with few adverse effects.

Histamine antagonists have not proved useful in asthma, although newer non-sedating antihistamines such as terfenadine may alleviate mild allergic asthma.

Problems with treatment

Failure to control asthma is often related to poor compliance with treatment regimens—for example, due to peer pressure in children. Compliance may also be poor when asthma is apparently controlled, so patients stop therapy (e.g. steroids, cromoglycate) because they are 'cured'. Poor inhaler techniques are common. Patient education and training is key to asthma therapy.

Severe uncontrolled asthma — 'status asthmaticus'

This requires immediate treatment and hospitalization. **Indications**: inability to complete sentences ('telegraph speaking'), high respiratory rate, tachycardia, PEFR <50% predicted.

Dangerously life-threatening when bradycardia/hypotension, cyanosis or coma/exhaustion are present and/or PEFR <30% predicted. **Treatment**: Immediate nebulized β_2-agonists delivered in oxygen and intravenous steroids, with subsequent oral prednisolone. In unresolving cases, intravenous β_2-agonists or xanthines and ventilation may be required.

23 Chronic obstructive pulmonary disease

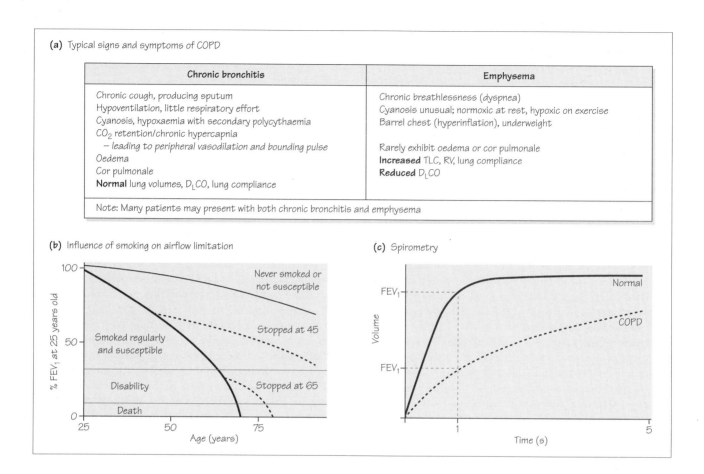

(a) Typical signs and symptoms of COPD

Chronic bronchitis	Emphysema
Chronic cough, producing sputum Hypoventilation, little respiratory effort Cyanosis, hypoxaemia with secondary polycythaemia CO_2 retention/chronic hypercapnia – leading to peripheral vasodilation and bounding pulse Oedema Cor pulmonale **Normal** lung volumes, D_LCO, lung compliance	Chronic breathlessness (dyspnea) Cyanosis unusual; normoxic at rest, hypoxic on exercise Barrel chest (hyperinflation), underweight Rarely exhibit oedema or cor pulmonale **Increased** TLC, RV, lung compliance **Reduced** D_LCO

Note: Many patients may present with both chronic bronchitis and emphysema

(b) Influence of smoking on airflow limitation

(c) Spirometry

Chronic obstructive pulmonary disease (COPD) is a group of chronic diseases characterized by reduced expiratory airflow and increased work of breathing. Other terms are COLD and COAD (chronic obstructive lung/airway disease). The reduced airflow can be due to decreased lung elastic recoil, increased airway resistance or both in combination. Typical patients show a progressive decline in lung function, interposed with intermittent **acute exacerbations**, eventually leading to progressive respiratory symptoms, disability and **respiratory failure** (Chapter 20). COPD encompasses **chronic bronchitis** and **emphysema,** which often present together (Fig. 23a). Asthma is generally not classified as COPD. Chronic hypoxaemia in COPD can lead to **pulmonary hypertension** (Chapter 24).

Pathogenesis: cigarette smoking is the single most important risk factor for development of COPD. Expiratory airflow normally decreases with age; cigarette smoking accelerates this decline (Fig. 23b). Other risk factors include increasing age, male gender, childhood respiratory infections, airway hyperreactivity, low socioeconomic status and α_1-antitrypsin deficiency (see Chapter 17).

COPD is **diagnosed** by airflow obstruction indicated by a **reduced FEV$_1$/FVC ratio** of <0.70 or FEV$_1$ two standard deviations below predicted provided restrictive disease is excluded (Fig. 23b; Chapter 18). Patients with COPD have symptoms of dysp-noea (breathlessness) at rest or on exertion. Many asymptomatic smokers have lung function abnormalities that predate symptoms, which may be prevented by early smoking cessation. Screening healthy smokers to identify subclinical airway obstruction is, however, controversial.

Chronic bronchitis is a clinical diagnosis requiring symptoms of chronic mucus hypersecretion. These symptoms include cough and excessive mucus production (associated with hypertrophy of mucus glands) for most days out of 3 months for ≥2 successive years, in the absence of airway tumour, acute/chronic infection or uncontrolled cardiac disease. Excessive airway mucus leads to increased airway resistance and obstruction. Most patients have normal total lung capacity (TLC), functional residual capacity (FRC), residual volume (RV), D_LCO (diffusing capacity) and static lung compliance (Chapter 18). Patients with advanced chronic bronchitis often fit into the '**blue bloater**' (type B non-fighter) morphology (see table), with marked **hypoxaemia, polycythaemia, CO_2 retention** and **cor pulmonale** (fluid retention/heart failure secondary to lung disease). Hypoxaemia is mostly due to V_A/Q mismatch (Chapter 14) and responds well to supplemental O_2. There are no radiographic signs diagnostic of chronic bronchitis.

Emphysema is caused by **progressive destruction of alveolar septa** and capillaries, leading to development of **enlarged airways**

and airspaces (bullae), **decreased lung elastic recoil** and **increased airway collapsibility**. The pathophysiology of emphysema may involve an imbalance between inflammatory cell proteases and antiprotease defences (Chapter 17). Centrilobular emphysema is associated with cigarette smoking and predominantly involves the upper lung zones. Panacinar emphysema is associated with α_1-antitrypsin deficiency (Chapter 17) and predominantly involves the lower lung zones. Patients with emphysema typically have airflow obstruction with elevated TLC, FRC and RV, reduced $D_L co$ and increased static lung compliance. Clinically, such patients tend towards the **'pink puffer'** (type A fighter) morphology, with **tachypnoea** and **dyspnoea** at rest, signs of hyperinflation and malnutrition including thin body and barrel chest, purse-lipped breathing using accessory muscles and distant breath sounds with a prolonged expiratory phase. Blood gases are normal at rest, with marked O_2 desaturation during exertion. Radiographically, emphysema may appear as hyperinflated lungs with a large retrosternal airspace and flat diaphragms. When the condition is advanced, there may be areas with a lack of vascularity or visualization of bullae. High-resolution computed tomography (CT) is useful to demonstrate enlarged airspaces and air trapping.

Therapy: there is no specific therapy to reverse COPD other than to prevent disease progression, minimize chronic symptoms and prevent acute exacerbations. Patients with advanced COPD may be candidates for lung transplantation. Lung volume reduction surgery has been reported to improve lung function in emphysema, but long-term efficacy and criteria for patient selection are under investigation.

Smoking cessation slows disease progression (Fig. 23b). Unfortunately, prolonged quit rates are usually <33%. The most effective program combines physician advice, nicotine replacement and antidepressant treatment. In α_1-antitrypsin deficiency, replacement therapy can increase plasma and lung antiprotease levels; however, the benefits on lung function and survival are controversial. O_2 **therapy** prolongs life in patients with resting daytime hypoxaemia by slowing progression of the disease. O_2 should be utilized as much as possible, as there is a dose relation with increasing time. Patients with nocturnal or exercise desaturation benefit from supplemental O_2 at night or during exercise. **Oral corticosteroids** (to reduce inflammation) improve function in <25% of COPD patients and due to the risk of side effects should not be used routinely without objective demonstration of benefit. Inhaled corticosteroids do not convincingly improve lung function.

Symptomatic therapy for COPD includes inhaled bronchodilators, theophylline, mucolytics and pulmonary rehabilitation. Beta-agonists and anticholinergics improve symptoms and lung function, possibly having additive effects when combined. Theophylline has negligible effects on spirometry, yet may improve exercise performance and blood gases. Patients producing large amounts of sputum may benefit from mucolytics. Pulmonary rehabilitation improves quality of life, exercise tolerance and hospitalizations without an effect on lung function.

Prevention of acute COPD exacerbations include pneumococcal and influenza vaccination. Patients with any combination of increased dyspnoea, increased sputum or purulent sputum benefit from antibiotics targeted against common respiratory pathogens (*Haemophilus influenzae*, *Moraxella catarrhalis*, *Streptococcus pneumoniae*). Short courses of oral corticosteroids improve lung function and hasten recovery in patients with acute exacerbations.

Overall prognosis for COPD patients is dependent on the severity of airflow obstruction. Patients with a FEV_1 <0.8 L have a yearly mortality of ~25%. Patients with cor pulmonale, hypercapnia, ongoing cigarette smoking and weight loss have a worse prognosis. Death usually occurs from infection, acute respiratory failure, pulmonary embolus or cardiac arrhythmia.

24 Pulmonary hypertension

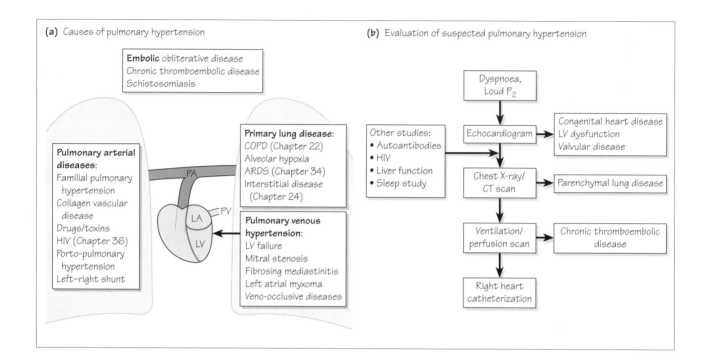

(a) Causes of pulmonary hypertension

Embolic obliterative disease
Chronic thromboembolic disease
Schistosomiasis

Pulmonary arterial diseases:
Familial pulmonary hypertension
Collagen vascular disease
Drugs/toxins
HIV (Chapter 36)
Porto-pulmonary hypertension
Left–right shunt

Primary lung disease:
COPD (Chapter 22)
Alveolar hypoxia
ARDS (Chapter 34)
Interstitial disease (Chapter 24)

Pulmonary venous hypertension:
LV failure
Mitral stenosis
Fibrosing mediastinitis
Left atrial myxoma
Veno-occlusive diseases

(b) Evaluation of suspected pulmonary hypertension

Dyspnoea, Loud P$_2$ → Echocardiogram → Congenital heart disease / LV dysfunction / Valvular disease

Other studies:
• Autoantibodies
• HIV
• Liver function
• Sleep study

Echocardiogram → Chest X-ray/CT scan → Parenchymal lung disease

Chest X-ray/CT scan → Ventilation/perfusion scan → Chronic thromboembolic disease

Ventilation/perfusion scan → Right heart catheterization

Pulmonary hypertension is defined as a mean pulmonary arterial (PA) pressure greater than **25 mmHg** at rest or during exercise. It is usually slow to develop and presents with non-specific symptoms, including dyspnoea on exertion, shortness of breath, palpitations, chest pain, light-headedness and syncope. Signs are difficult to elicit early and may only include an increased pulmonic component of the second heart sound. With more severe hypertension, **right ventricular dysfunction** will be apparent, including jugular venous distension, right ventricular heave, pedal oedema and hepatic enlargement. Patients with pulmonary hypertension usually die from **progressive right heart failure** (see the section on heart failure in *The Cardiovascular System at a Glance,* Chapter 43). Detection of pulmonary hypertension requires a high index of suspicion, since signs and symptoms are non-specific and the diagnosis requires further testing.

Since PA pressure is a function of **pulmonary vascular resistance**, cardiac output and back-pressure (left atrial pressure), many kinds of abnormality can result in pulmonary hypertension (Fig. 24a). Increased left atrial (LA) pressure, most commonly due to left ventricular dysfunction as in **congestive heart failure**, leads to elevation of PA pressure by increasing back-pressure through the lungs. **Mitral insufficiency** or **stenosis** may also increase PA pressure enough to cause hypertension. In these cases, patients will often have signs of pulmonary capillary hypertension such as crackles. Echocardiography should demonstrate LA enlargement.

Increases in pulmonary vascular resistance may occur in the veins, capillaries or arteries. Increases in **capillary resistance** are common and may occur in any lung disease that causes capillary distortion or reduction in surface area. **Interstitial lung diseases**

(Chapter 27) such as pulmonary fibrosis, scleroderma or sarcoidosis cause capillary distortion, as lung parenchyma is affected. Destruction of capillaries occurs in emphysema (Chapter 23) or pneumonectomy. **Arterial resistance** may increase due to vasospasm, remodeling or mechanical obstruction. **Alveolar hypoxia** is a potent stimulus for arterial vasoconstriction and may cause pulmonary hypertension in COPD or other chronic lung diseases (Chapter 23), or at high altitude. Remodeling of pulmonary arterioles is characteristic of idiopathic pulmonary arterial vasculopathy (**PAV**, formerly termed **primary pulmonary hypertension**), but may also be seen in **chronic hypoxia** and chronic **left-to-right shunting** due to congenital heart disease. PAV may be due to chronic arterial vasospasm, as some patients demonstrate a reduction in PA pressure after administration of vasodilators (e.g. diltiazem or prostacyclin). Acute and chronic venous thromboembolism causes pulmonary hypertension by mechanical obstruction of the pulmonary arterial bed. In acute thromboembolism, a component of vasospasm is also present, as the platelet-rich thromboembolus releases vasoactive mediators such as thromboxane, serotonin or platelet activating factor. **Abnormalities of pulmonary veins** are an uncommon cause of pulmonary hypertension, but may occur in pulmonary veno-occlusive disease or in fibrosing mediastinitis secondary to chronic histoplasmosis or **tuberculosis** (Chapter 33).

Increases in cardiac output alone seldom cause pulmonary hypertension, as the lungs have a large capacity to accommodate increases in flow through recruitment and distension of the pulmonary vasculature. Up to two-thirds of normal lung can be removed (increasing flow through the remaining lung by three times) before pulmonary hypertension will develop. However, chronic elevations of cardiac output (e.g. congenital cardiac defects, hyperthyroidism) may cause pulmonary hypertension, as the chronic high flow causes arterial remodelling and increased resistance.

Evaluation

Evaluation of patients with suspected pulmonary hypertension (Fig. 24b) begins with **echocardiography**, allowing calculation of right ventricular systolic pressure and visualization of left atrium, mitral valve, right ventricle and congenital abnormalities. If pulmonary hypertension is found in conjunction with an enlarged LA, it is most likely due to either left ventricular or mitral disease. Chest radiology, pulmonary function testing and measurement of arterial oxygen allow detection of parenchymal disease or hypoxia. In the absence of LA enlargement or pulmonary parenchymal disease, further evaluation of pulmonary arteries is necessary. Ventilation/perfusion scanning is most useful to demonstrate chronic thromboemboli. **Right heart catheterization** is the definitive test for the assessment of pulmonary hypertension, as PA pressure can be measured directly and LA pressure estimated from the pulmonary capillary wedge pressure (see *The Cardiovascular System at a Glance,* Chapter 32).

Patients with pulmonary hypertension without an elevated LA pressure and no apparent pulmonary venous, lung parenchymal, chronic thromboemboli or congenital heart disease are assumed to have PAV. PAV is most often idiopathic, but may be associated with autoimmune diseases such as scleroderma. There is a familial form of PAV with autosomal dominant inheritance and associations between PAV and use of anorexigenic drugs.

Treatment

Patients with pulmonary hypertension die of **right heart failure**; severe right heart failure with right atrial pressure >20 mmHg has a 1-year mortality greater than 75%. Therefore therapy for pulmonary hypertension in most patients is directed at the underlying abnormality, to relieve right ventricular strain. There is generally no specific therapy for pulmonary hypertension in cases of left ventricular dysfunction, pulmonary venous disease or pulmonary parenchymal diseases. Hypoxaemic patients with parenchymal lung disease benefit from O_2 therapy to diminish hypoxic vasoconstriction. Patients with **thromboembolic disease** (Chapter 25) should receive anticoagulation and evaluation for surgical thromboembolectomy. Patients with PAV should also receive **anticoagulation** to prevent microthrombi or the devastating effect of an acute thromboembolus (Chapter 25). PAV is the only disease where therapy directed at the pulmonary arterial abnormality has been shown to benefit. Most patients with PAV require chronic infusions or frequent nebulization of **prostacyclin** to improve survival. Prostacyclin has acute vasodilator properties, but an effect on pulmonary vascular remodelling or endothelial function more likely explains its positive effect on patient long-term function and survival. New therapies including endothelin antagonists or nitric oxide are under investigation. Lung transplantation may be considered for patients with pulmonary hypertension due to parenchymal lung disease or PAV.

25 Venous thromboembolism and pulmonary embolism

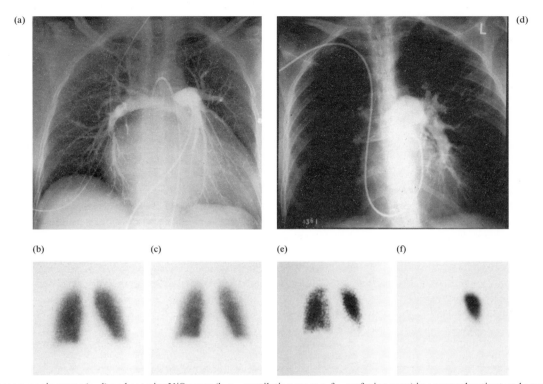

Fig. 25 Pulmonary angiograms (a, d) and anterior V/Q scans (b, e — ventilation scan; c, f — perfusion scan) in a normal patient and a patient with a massive pulmonary embolism. The angiogram (d) shows complete block of the right pulmonary artery (compare with a). This is reflected by the loss of right lung perfusion (f), but not ventilation (e).

Table 1 Risk factors for venous thromboembolism and pulmonary embolism.

Virchow's triad of venous stasis, hypercoaguability, and vascular injury are predictors of increased risk for DVT/PE			
General	**Trauma** e.g.	**Low flow states** e.g.	**Inherited deficiencies in:**
Smoking	Surgery (e.g. hip/knee replacement)	Chronic heart disease	Protein S, Protein C
Pregnancy	Spinal cord injury	Immobilization	Antithrombin III, Plasminogen
Oral contraceptives			Antiphospholipid antibodies
Age	**Disease** e.g.	**Damage to endothelium** e.g.	**Other inherited:**
Obesity	Malignancy	Prior thrombosis	Resistance to protein C (factor V Leiden)
	Nephrotic syndrome	Intravascular catheters	Prothrombin variant 20210
		Atherosclerosis	Hyperhomocysteinaemia

NB Risk factors add together in a cumulative fashion.

Venous thromboembolism and its most significant complication, **pulmonary embolism (PE)**, are common clinical disorders that have a substantial impact on patient morbidity and mortality; Table 1 shows risk factors. PE is most often a complication of **deep venous thrombosis (DVT)**. Both disorders usually present with non-specific signs or symptoms, and are commonly underdiagnosed; they therefore require an appropriate clinical suspicion and a systematic diagnostic approach.

Deep venous thrombosis

Nearly all clinically significant cases of PE arise from DVT in the lower extremities and pelvis. These thrombi typically originate below the knee. Approximately 15–25% will propagate proximally to the femoral and iliac arteries and have a 50% risk of embolizing to the lung. Thrombi may develop in the axillary and subclavian veins, usually due to surgery or intravenous catheters, but these are usually smaller, with less risk of catastrophic consequences if they embolize. Soon after thrombus formation, the intrinsic fibrinolytic cascade begins to organize the thrombus. The risk of a thrombus embolizing is greatest early during ongoing proliferation and decreases once it is organized.

Pulmonary embolism

When a thrombus embolizes to the lung, respiratory or circulatory

Table 2 Strategies for prophylaxis against DVT.

Risk of DVT	Patient	Regimen
Low (<1%)	<40 years Minor surgery (<1 h) Minimal immobility	Early ambulation Compression stockings
Moderate (5–10%)	>40 years General surgery (>1 h) Cardiac, medical condition Cerebrovascular accident ? Inherited hypercoagulability	Low-dose: Unfractionated heparin or Low molecular weight heparin
High (>15%)	Extended surgery Knee/hip joint Hip fracture Trauma	Full-dose: Low molecular weight heparin Warfarin (Coumadin)

abnormalities occur due to sudden occlusion of a pulmonary artery or arteriole. Occlusion of regional perfusion causes an increase in dead space, necessitating an **increase in minute ventilation** to maintain normal $P_a\text{CO}_2$. Surfactant production in the lung region distal to the embolus may be reduced after 24 h, resulting in **atelectasis**. Most patients with PE have **hypoxaemia** or a wide A–a gradient, mostly due to V_A/Q **mismatching** (Chapter 13). **Pulmonary infarction** occurs in less than 25% of cases of PE. Circulatory complications arise from obliteration of the pulmonary vascular bed and a reduction of cardiac output. The severity of complications is related to the amount of lung embolized and the pre-existing state of the pulmonary vasculature and right ventricle (RV); a single large embolus can be catastrophic, whereas multiple small emboli can cause 'pruning' of the smaller arteries. **Compensatory mechanisms** to maintain cardiac output include pulmonary vascular distension and recruitment, increased heart rate, catecholamine-induced increased venous return and RV contractility. With >50% obstruction circulatory collapse may occur. Less severe emboli may be fatal to patients with pre-existing lung or heart disease.

Signs and symptoms

The **signs and symptoms** of DVT/PE are non-specific. Lower extremity pain, swelling, erythema and Homan's sign (pain in the calf on dorsiflexion of the foot) occur in a minority of patients with DVT. Most patients with PE have **dyspnoea, pleuritic chest pain, apprehension** and **tachypnoea**. Tachycardia, cough, crackles, haemoptysis, diaphoresis, syncope and chest pain are less common. With severe PE, signs related to **RV failure** (e.g. hypotension, jugular venous distension) may occur. Most patients with PE have non-specific abnormalities on chest X-ray, including atelectasis or small effusions. Non-specific electrocardiographic (ECG) abnormalities are common; with RV strain, the ECG may show an $S_1Q_3T_3$ pattern, right axis deviation (RAD) or right bundle-branch block (RBBB). **Arterial blood gas abnormalities** are very common, usually consisting of **widened A–a gradient, hypoxaemia** and **hypocapnia** (despite increased dead space). None of these tests will diagnose PE; however, their results may be useful in assessing clinical likelihood.

Diagnosis

Deep venography or **pulmonary angiography** are the diagnostic

standard, although **V/Q scanning** is usually the initial test for assessment of PE, as it is non-invasive, safe and clinically useful (Fig. 25; see Chapter 19). A negative perfusion scan effectively rules out PE and a 'high probability' scan (multiple segmental perfusion defects with normal ventilation) has a >85% probability of PE (Fig. 25). With a high clinical suspicion, a high-probability V/Q scan has a positive predictive value >95%. Unfortunately, most V/Q scans are non-diagnostic or indeterminate, with a 15–50% likelihood of PE, necessitating further diagnostic testing. **Non-invasive imaging** of the lower extremity deep veins with Doppler imaging or impedance plethysmography is useful, since the presence of thrombosis requires treatment similar to PE. In patients with underlying cardiac or pulmonary disease, **pulmonary angiography** is indicated if the above tests are not diagnostic. In patients with no underlying cardiac or pulmonary disease, **serial lower extremity imaging** may be performed and treatment withheld in the absence of a positive result. A negative d-dimer assay may be useful to rule out DVT/PE. **Spiral/helical computed tomography** (CT) has been found to have a sensitivity for PE of 70–95% (higher for more proximal emboli) and a specificity >90% when interpreted by experienced readers. CT scanning also allows visualization of parenchymal abnormalities and may be particularly useful in patients with chronic obstructive pulmonary disease (COPD) or extensive chest X-ray abnormalities, where V/Q scanning is often indeterminate. **Echocardiography** may reveal RV dysfunction in PE and rule out **pericardial tamponade** or severe left ventricular (LV) dysfunction. **Transoesophageal echocardiography** may visualize thromboemboli in the main pulmonary arteries, but not in the lobar or segmental arteries.

Prevention in patients at risk

Depending on the level of risk (low, medium or high) prophylaxis with pneumatic compression devices, low-dose aspirin or heparin, adjusted-dose heparin, low molecular weight heparin or warfarin are effective (Table 2).

Treatment

The cornerstone of therapy for DVT/PE is **anticoagulation**, which stops propagation of existing thrombus and allows organization. Therapy should be instituted immediately to patients with a high suspicion of disease, because further embolization may be life-threatening. **Unfractionated heparin (UFH)** or **low molecular weight heparin (LMWH)** for 5–7 days, followed by **warfarin** for 6 months, is standard therapy. UFH and warfarin must be monitored, as subtherapeutic effects increase the risk of recurrent thromboembolism. LMWH is more bioavailable and does not require monitoring. Patients with inherited or acquired hypercoagulability may require lifelong therapy. Patients with contraindications to anticoagulation (recent surgery, haemorrhagic stroke, central nervous system metastases, active bleeding) or recurrent PE while on therapeutic anticoagulation should receive an **inferior vena cava (IVC) filter** to prevent fatal PE.

Although activation of **fibrinolysis** with **thrombolytics** hastens resolution of perfusion defects and RV dysfunction, there is lack of convincing evidence for benefit. Moreover, thrombolytics cause increased bleeding complications, including a 0.3–1.5% risk of intracerebral haemorrhage. Therefore thrombolytics are only recommended for life-threatening PE with compromised haemodynamics.

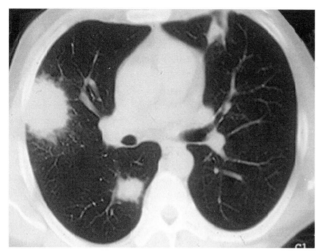

Fig. 26.1 CT scan of patient with Wegener's granulomatosis, showing large cavitating masses.

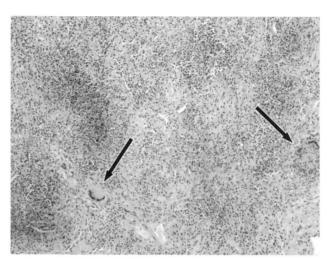

Fig. 26.2 Histological section showing necrobiotic regions with multinucleate giant cells (arrows).

Since the entire cardiac output traverses the lung through the pulmonary circulation, it is not surprising that a variety of disorders characterized by **vascular inflammation** involve the lung, although such pulmonary vasculitis is relatively uncommon. These disorders may be secondary to systemic collagen vascular disease — such as **rheumatoid arthritis, scleroderma** or **systemic lupus erythematosus (SLE)** — or **primary vasculitides** that involve pulmonary blood vessels (**Wegener's granulomatosis, microscopic polyangiitis, lymphomatoid granulomatosis, allergic granulomatosis** and **angiitis**). Antiglomerular basement membrane disease (**Goodpasture's syndrome**), while not a vasculitis, is included, since its clinical presentation may be similar to that of pulmonary vasculitis. Most of these disorders cause systemic symptoms and depending on the blood vessel involved may cause pulmonary infiltrates, masses or alveolar haemorrhage.

Collagen vascular diseases

Rheumatoid arthritis may cause vasculitis and **pulmonary hypertension** (Chapter 24); however, this complication is far less frequent than pleural disease (Chapter 28) or diffuse parenchymal disease (Chapter 27). Patients may develop **Caplan's syndrome** as a result of dust inhalation (e.g. coal dust) (Chapter 31). **Limited cutaneous scleroderma** often spares lung parenchyma and causes pulmonary hypertension by direct involvement of the pulmonary arterioles. While not common, **pulmonary capillaritis** causing alveolar haemorrhage due to **SLE** is a devastating complication of the disease with a high mortality rate. Patients generally have a pre-existing diagnosis of SLE, usually with renal involvement. Rarely, SLE may cause pulmonary hypertension by direct involvement of the pulmonary vasculature. Clinically, this is indistinguishable from pulmonary arterial hypertension (Chapter 24).

Granulomatoses

Wegener's granulomatosis (WG) is a systemic vasculitis that predominantly involves the upper and lower respiratory systems and the renal glomeruli. The vascular inflammation may involve arterioles, capillaries and venules. Patients are generally aged 40–60 and present with upper respiratory symptoms usually involving the sinuses (sinusitis) or nasopharynx (ulcers, septal perforation, saddle nose deformity). Radiographic abnormalities in the chest are common, even in the absence of cough or haemoptysis. Most commonly, they appear as nodules or masses, often with cavitation (Fig. 26.1), but they may appear as parenchymal infiltrates. Renal disease is usual and consists of glomerulonephritis with haematuria, proteinuria and red blood cell (RBC) casts. The c-ANCA (antiproteinase 3; **antineutrophil cytoplasmic antibody**) has a 60–90% sensitivity and >90% specificity for WG. Transbronchial lung biopsies are seldom sufficient to diagnose WG. Larger amounts of parenchyma from open or thoracoscopic biopsy are necessary to demonstrate granulomatous inflammation in arterial walls or perivascular spaces. Biopsies of the paranasal sinuses or kidneys may also be diagnostic in the proper clinical context. WG may also involve the ears (otitis media), eyes (conjunctivitis, uveitis), heart (coronary arteries), peripheral nervous system, skin or joints.

Microscopic polyangiitis (MPA) is also a vasculitis of small vessels, which has microscopic similarities to WG and polyarteritis nodosa. In contrast to WG, MPA does not involve the nasopharynx and sinuses and is usually associated with p-ANCA (antimyeloperoxidase) rather than c-ANCA. It is often seen in patients with hepatitis B or C infection. **Treatment** with corticosteroids and cyclophosphamide substantially reduces mortality.

Lymphomatoid granulomatosis (LG) is a systemic vasculitis of the lungs, kidneys, central nervous system (CNS) and skin. LG

Table 1 Pulmonary vasculitides.

Disease	Blood vessel	Comment
Collagen vascular diseases		
Rheumatoid arthritis	Arteries/arterioles	Uncommon
Scleroderma	Fibrosis in arterioles	CREST syndrome
SLE	Capillaritis	Pulmonary hemorrhage
Vasculitides		
Wegener's granulomatosis	Granulomatous inflammation	Pulmonary hemorrhage common
	Arteriolar/venular vasculitis	c-ANCA (90%)
	Fibrinoid necrosis	
	Capillaritis (1/3)	
Microscopic polyangiitis	Arteriole/venule vasculitis	Related to Wegener's and PAN
	Capillaritis, fibrinoid necrosis	p-ANCA, hepatitis B, C
Lymphomatoid granulomatosis	Angiocentric/angiodestructive lymphocytes,	Epstein–Barr Virus
	plasma cells, atypical lymphocytes	Lymphoproliferative
Allergic granulomatosis and angiitis	Necrotizing vasculitis in small and	Asthma, eosinophilia
	medium-sized arteries, arterioles, venules	66% p-ANCA or c-ANCA
	Granulomas, eosinophils	
	Fibrinoid necrosis	
Anti-GBM disease	Intra-alveolar haemorrhage	Smoking, recent infection
	Linear IgG in basement membrane	
	Minimal inflammation	

ANCA, antineutrophil cytoplasmic antibody; CREST, calcinosis, Raynaud's phenomenon, esophageal involvement, sclerodactyly and telangiectasia; GBM, glomerular basement membrane; PAN, polyarteritis nodosa; SLE, systemic lupus erythematosus.

is strongly associated with, and may be a late complication of, Epstein–Barr virus (EBV) infection. It behaves like an indolent lymphoproliferative disease and may transform into a B-cell lymphoma. Patients typically have fever, malaise, cough, dyspnoea and a papular rash. Radiographic abnormalities usually consist of multiple lower lobe nodular densities. Lung biopsy shows angiocentric/angiodestructive mixed cell infiltration with lymphocytes, plasma cells and atypical lymphocytes. Vascular occlusion and necrosis are common. LG is considered to be a lymphoproliferative disorder and is treated with chemotherapy and corticosteroids. Without treatment, the disease progresses and is usually fatal.

Allergic granulomatosis and angiitis (Churg–Strauss syndrome) is a medium/small vessel granulomatous vasculitis of the lung, skin, heart, nervous system and kidney. It is probably the second most common pulmonary vasculitis after WG. Most patients have a history of allergic rhinitis and/or asthma and peripheral eosinophilia that may predate the vasculitis by up to a decade. Patients will present with worsening asthma, fever, malaise, subcutaneous tender nodules, mononeuritis multiplex and radiographic infiltrates. There may also be pericarditis, abdominal pain and glomerulonephritis. Radiographic abnormalities are most often patchy, fleeting infiltrates, but may include cavitating nodules or masses, interstitial infiltrates or pleural effusions. Chest computed tomography (CT) may show ground glass opacities or peribronchial thickening. p-ANCA or c-ANCA may be positive. Lung biopsy will show perivascular granulomatous inflammation, small artery and vein vasculitis, prominent eosinophils and necrosis. The diagnosis may be made without biopsy in the presence of asthma, eosinophilia, migratory pulmonary infiltrates and neuropathy. Most patients respond to corticosteroids. Cyclophosphamide or azathioprine may be added in resistant cases. Patients who respond to therapy seldom relapse. Patients with an onset of asthma immediately before or concurrent with vasculitis have a poorer prognosis. Overall, the survival is >70%, with mortality usually due to cardiac, CNS, renal or gastrointestinal involvement.

Anti-glomerular basement membrane (GBM) disease is caused by antibodies directed against the glomerular membranes causing glomerulonephritis. In **Goodpasture's syndrome** these antibodies sometimes cross-react with alveolar basement membrane, causing alveolar haemorrhage. Alveolar haemorrhage seems to occur predominantly in patients who smoke cigarettes, or who have a recent respiratory infection which may alter alveolar permeability. Patients present with rapidly progressive glomerulonephritis, haemoptysis, anaemia and diffuse alveolar infiltrates on radiographs. In contrast to the primary vasculitides, prolonged systemic symptoms such as fever, malaise or rash are uncommon. Pulmonary function testing demonstrates elevated $D_L\text{CO}$ from extravasated haemoglobin in the lung. Serial measurement of $D_L\text{CO}$ may show a decline as extravascular haemoglobin saturates with CO. Diagnosis requires demonstration of anti-GBM antibodies in serum or linear IgG in glomerular or alveolar basement membranes. c-ANCA or p-ANCA may be positive. Patients with Goodpasture's syndrome should be treated with plasmapheresis, cyclophosphamide and corticosteroids. Therapy may control alveolar haemorrhage; however, renal disease is usually irreversible if the presenting creatinine is >5 mg/dL.

27 Interstitial lung disease

Causes of interstitial lung diseases			
Primary/predominantly respiratory disease	Autoimmune and collagen vascular disease	Drugs and therapies	Occupational/enviromental (see Chapter 31)

Acute eosinophilic pneumonia
Acute interstitial pneumonia
  (Hamman–Rich syndrome)
Cryptogenic organizing pneumonia
Eosinophilic granuloma
Idiopathic pulmonary fibrosis
Lymphangiolyomyomatosis
Lymphangitic carcinomatosis
Lymphocytic interstitial pneumonia
Sarcoidosis
	Ankylosing spondylitis
	Dermatomyositis/polymyositis
	Rheumatoid arthritis
	Scleroderma
	Systemic lupus erythematosus
	Sjögren's syndrome
		Amiodarone
		Bleomycin
		Cyclophosphamide
		Gold
		Methotrexate
		Nitrofurantoin
		Oxygen
		Penicillamine
		Radiation
			Asbestosis
			Berylliosis
			Coal worker's pneumoconiosis
			Farmer's lung
			Hard metal disease
			Extrinsic allergic alveolitis
			  (hypersensitivity pneumonitis)
			Pigeon fancier's lung
			Silicosis

(a) Cellular basis of fibrosis (not to scale)

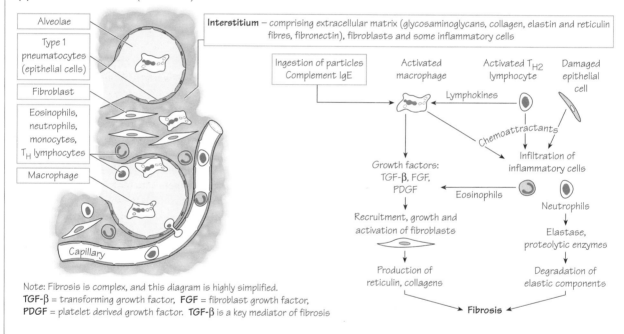

Alveolae

Type 1 pneumatocytes (epithelial cells)

Fibroblast

Eosinophils, neutrophils, monocytes, T$_H$ lymphocytes

Macrophage

Capillary

Interstitium – comprising extracellular matrix (glycosaminoglycans, collagen, elastin and reticulin fibres, fibronectin), fibroblasts and some inflammatory cells

Ingestion of particles Complement IgE

Activated macrophage

Activated T$_{H2}$ lymphocyte

Damaged epithelial cell

Lymphokines

Chemoattractants

Growth factors: TGF-β, FGF, PDGF

Eosinophils

Infiltration of inflammatory cells

Neutrophils

Recruitment, growth and activation of fibroblasts

Elastase, proteolytic enzymes

Production of reticulin, collagens

Degradation of elastic components

Fibrosis

Note: Fibrosis is complex, and this diagram is highly simplified.
TGF-β = transforming growth factor, **FGF** = fibroblast growth factor,
PDGF = platelet derived growth factor. **TGF-β** is a key mediator of fibrosis

(b) CT scan showing typical honeycomb lung appearance and interstitial infiltrates with some dorsal consolidation

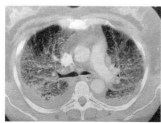

(c) CXR of patient with sarcoidosis (see text)

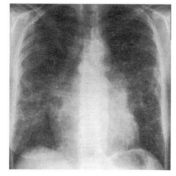

(d) CT scan of sarcoidosis

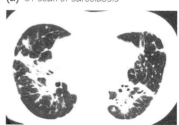

Interstitial lung disease (ILD) refers to an extensive variety of acute and chronic clinical disorders, characterized by inflammation or fibrosis of alveolar–capillary units and distal airways (Fig. 27a). These diseases are not limited to the interstitium, but may involve all of the matrix components of the lung, such that 'diffuse parenchymal lung diseases' is a more accurate description of their morphology. The symptoms of ILD are most often **dyspnoea** and **cough**, usually indolent over months. Signs include **digital clubbing** and **diffuse inspiratory crackles**. With advanced disease, there may be **hypoxaemia** and right ventricular failure. Pulmonary function tests (Chapter 18) reveal reduced total lung capacity (TLC), functional residual capacity (FRC) and residual volume (**RV**) due to **decreased compliance** and **increased elastic recoil** of the lungs. $D_L co$ is reduced because of a reduction in surface area for gas exchange secondary to reduced lung volume. With exercise, there is rapid shallow breathing and O_2 desaturation. Most (>90%) of patients with ILD will have an **abnormal chest X-ray**, with any combination or alveolar, interstitial or mixed infiltrates, typically predominating in the lower lobes. Small (0.5–2 cm), thick-walled cysts denote advanced fibrosis and give rise to a typical radiological appearance known as '**honeycomb lung**' (Fig. 27b). High-resolution computed tomography (HRCT) allows a far more accurate distinction of parenchymal involvement and may have diagnostic or therapeutic implications. **Bronchoalveolar lavage (BAL)** may be useful to diagnose malignancy, eosinophilic pneumonia, alveolar proteinosis or alveolar haemorrhage. BAL fluid containing increased inflammatory cells (Chapter 17) reflects alveolitis and correlates with ground glass infiltrates on HRCT; this may identify patients with rapidly progressive or potentially reversible disease. **Open** or **thoracoscopic lung biopsy** is usually necessary to determine a diagnosis and therapeutic plan.

ILD may be classified clinically or histologically. Clinically, ILD may be caused by occupational or environmental exposures (Chapter 31), drugs/therapies, autoimmune diseases and primary pulmonary conditions or may be idiopathic (see Table). Histological patterns include usual interstitial pneumonia (UIP), desquamative interstitial pneumonia (DIP), non-specific interstitial pneumonia (NSIP), acute interstitial pneumonitis (AIP, Hamman–Rich syndrome), lymphocytic interstitial pneumonia (LIP), organizing pneumonia, eosinophilic pneumonia, granulomatous disease or honeycomb lung. The histological patterns are usually not disease-specific. Knowledge of clinical and histological associations is necessary to diagnose and treat these disorders.

Idiopathic pulmonary fibrosis (IPF)/cryptogenic fibrosing alveolitis (CFA) typically occurs in men in their 60s, with subpleural fibrosis in the lower lobes. UIP is the most common histological pattern of IPF/CFA, although it may represent a point in the progression of DIP or NSIP to end-stage honeycomb lung. UIP is a patchy disease with areas of normal lung, interstitial inflammation and fibrosis with fibroblast proliferation (Fig. 27a). The median survival in patients with UIP is less than 5 years and corticosteroids have minimal effect. DIP and NSIP are diagnosed at younger ages, have more diffuse, more cellular, less fibrotic involvement and respond well to corticosteroids. The mean survival in patients with DIP and NSIP is >10 years and complete recovery is attainable with therapy. These differences highlight the utility of histological examination of the lungs in patients with clinical IPF/CFA.

Sarcoidosis is a multiorgan granulomatous disease of unknown aetiology, but with characteristic clinical and pathologic features. Activated CD4 lymphocytes appear to participate in the pathophysiology. Sarcoidosis is usually asymptomatic, presenting with unsuspected bilateral hilar adenopathy on X-ray in young (20–40 years) people. Symptomatic sarcoidosis most often involves the lung with ILD, but may also be present in the eyes, skin, joints, central nervous system (CNS), heart or liver. Radiographically, lung disease manifests as any combination of hilar/paratracheal adenopathy, reticulonodular infiltrates or advanced fibrosis with cysts (Fig. 27c). Pleural disease is uncommon. Patients with significant radiographic parenchymal abnormalities may have a normal chest physical examination. The classic histological feature of sarcoidosis is **non-caseating granulomas**, which are commonly found on transbronchial biopsy even in the absence of radiographic abnormalities. **Angiotensin-converting enzyme** is commonly elevated in sarcoidosis, but this test is neither sensitive nor specific for diagnostic purposes. Sarcoidosis is usually a self-limited disease without therapy. Up to 50% of cases resolve without treatment within 3 years; however, some patients will develop progressive ILD involvement. Patients should be followed with periodic radiographs and pulmonary function tests. Therapy is indicated for significant organ involvement or significant impairment on pulmonary function testing. Oral corticosteroids are standard therapy and most patients achieve remission within months. The optimal duration of therapy is uncertain and is individualized for each patient. Immunosuppressive or immunomodulatory medications have been reported to benefit selected patients, but no controlled trial has demonstrated superiority over corticosteroids. Lung transplantation is an option for patients with advanced fibrosis.

Interstitial lung disease is a common complication of **autoimmune** or **collagen vascular diseases** such as scleroderma, rheumatoid arthritis, systemic lupus erythematosus (**SLE**), polymyositis/dermatomyositis (**PM/DM**) and *Sjögren's syndrome*. It is important to distinguish this manifestation of the underlying disease from a complication of drug therapy or opportunistic infection. These patients have signs, symptoms, radiographs and pulmonary function tests similar to patients with IPF/CFA or AIP. Some patients with symptomatic disease will respond to aggressive therapy with chemotherapeutic agents plus corticosteroids. Up to 70% of patients with **scleroderma** may have interstitial fibrosis clinically or radiographically. Patients with a ground-glass pattern on HRCT or alveolitis on BAL have more rapid deterioration of lung function. The median survival of 8 years is better than that in patients with IPF/CFA. Interstitial lung disease is also common in patients with rheumatoid arthritis, with males, smokers and patients with severe joint disease at higher risk. Acute and chronic interstitial pneumonitis occurs in <10% of patients with SLE. While PM/DM is an uncommon disease, up to 50% of patients will develop interstitial lung disease and it is a frequent cause of mortality. Interstitial disease is often associated with the presence of **antisynthetase autoantibodies** (e.g. anti-Jo-1). LIP is the most common interstitial lung disease in *Sjögren's syndrome* and may evolve to **pulmonary lymphoma**.

Causes of pleural effusions

Exudative:		
(protein ratio pleural/serum >0.5 **or** LDH ratio pleural/serum >0.6 **or** pleural LDH >0.66 of top normal serum value)		
Infectious	**Autoimmune/collagen vascular**	**Miscellaneous**
Para-pneumonic	Systemic lupus erythematosus	Pulmonary embolism
• aerobic bacterial pneumonia	Rheumatoid arthritis	Drug reactions
• anaerobic bacterial pneumonia	**Neoplastic**	Asbestos exposure
Empyema		Haemothorax
Tuberculosis	Lung cancer	Chylothorax
Parasitic	Metastatic disease	Post-cardiac
• amoeba	Mesothelioma	surgery
• echinococcus	**Abdominal**	Post-myocardial
• paragonimus		infarction
Viral	Pancreatitis/pseudocyst	Meig's syndrome
	Oesophageal rupture	
	Liver abscess	
	Splenic abscess	
Transudative: (meets none of the criteria for exudate)		
	Cirrhosis/hepatic hydrothorax Nephrotic disease	
	Congestive heart failure Peritoneal dialysis	
	Myxoedema	

CXR of effusion in left lung

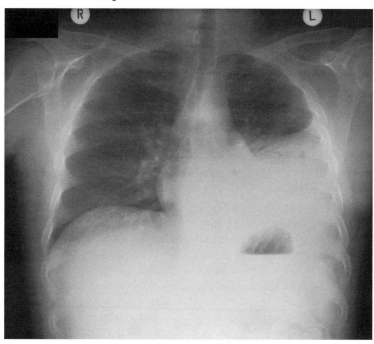

The potential space between the **parietal** and **visceral pleurae** serves as a coupling system between the lung and the chest wall, and normally contains a small amount of fluid. A negative pleural pressure is maintained by the dynamic tension between the chest wall and the lung (Chapter 3). Both pleurae have a systemic blood supply and lymphatics, although lymphatic drainage of the pleural space is predominantly via the parietal pleura. Fluid flux through the pleural space is determined by Starling's relationship between microvascular pressures, oncotic pressures, permeability and surface area. Normally, there is net filtration of **transudative** (protein-poor) fluid into the pleural space that is balanced by resorption via the parietal lymphatics. **Pneumothorax** is an important condition that occurs when air enters the pleural space and pleural pressure rises to atmospheric pressure; it is discussed in detail in Chapter 29. **Chylothorax** is due to accumulation of triglyceride-rich lymph in the pleural space, generally as the result of damage to the thoracic duct causing leakage into the pleural space, for example due to trauma or carcinoma. **Empyema** is accumulation of pus. **Pleurisy** is a term commonly used to describe the sharp localized pain arising from any disease of the pleura. It is made worse by deep inspiration and coughing.

Most diseases of the pleura present with **pleural effusion**. Effusions are due to excessive fluid formation or inadequate fluid clearance. Symptoms develop if the fluid is **inflammatory** or if **pulmonary mechanics** are compromised. Thus, the most common symptoms of a pleural effusion are **pleuritic chest pain**, **dull aching pain**, **fullness of the chest** or **dyspnoea**. Physical examination reveals decreased breath sounds, dullness to percussion, decreased tactile or vocal fremitus. If there is inflammation, there may be a friction rub. **Compressive atelectasis** may cause bronchial breath sounds.

Pathophysiology: it is useful to categorize pleural effusions as **transudative** or **exudative** (Fig. 28a). **Transudative effusions** are usually due to an imbalance in Starling's forces across normal pleural membranes, have protein-poor fluid, are often bilateral and are not associated with fever, pleuritic pain or tenderness to palpation. The most common cause of a transudative effusion is **congestive heart failure**. Other causes include cirrhosis with ascites, nephrotic syndrome, pericardial disease or peritoneal dialysis.

Exudative effusions imply disease of the pleura or the adjacent lung and are characterized by an increased protein, lactate dehydrogenase (LDH), cholesterol or white blood cell count (WBC) (Fig. 28a). The differential diagnosis of exudative effusions is broad, including: infection, malignancy, autoimmune disease, oesophageal perforation and pancreatitis.

The diagnostic evaluation of a pleural effusion should include measurement of cell count with differential, pH, protein, LDH, cholesterol and glucose. These studies will usually distinguish exudates from transudates and will often suggest a specific diagnosis.

For example, extremely low glucose is typical for empyema, malignancy, tuberculosis (Chapter 33), rheumatoid arthritis, systemic lupus erythematosus (SLE) or oesophageal perforation. If clinically indicated, a specific diagnosis may be obtained from microbiologic stains and culture, cytopathology, amylase, triglycerides and measurement of antinuclear antibody (ANA) titre. Although all patients with SLE have a positive ANA titre in the pleural fluid, it is also present in a significant proportion (~15%) of other effusions; these may be related to malignancy.

Pneumonia (Chapter 32) commonly causes parapneumonic pleural effusions. These effusions are usually sterile exudates with a neutrophilic leukocytosis and require only treatment of the pneumonia to resolve. However, if bacteria invade the pleural space, a complicated parapneumonic effusion or empyema will develop. These effusions are characterized by a low pH and extensive fibrin deposition causing fluid loculation and require adequate open or closed drainage for healing. *Streptococcus pneumoniae, Staphylococcus aureus,* Gram-negative bacteria and anaerobes commonly cause complicated effusions.

Tuberculosis pleurisy occurs when a subpleural focus of primary infection ruptures into the pleural space, causing a delayed hypersensitivity response. Subsequently, an exudative effusion with a lymphocytic leukocytosis, a paucity of macrophages and an elevated adenosine deaminase will develop. Patients develop fever, dyspnoea, pleuritic pain and a positive tuberculin response (see Chapter 33). Granulomatous inflammation is seen on pleural biopsy and culture of pleural tissue has the highest diagnostic yield.

Primary lung malignancies or **metastases** to the lung may cause pleural effusions by direct invasion or by obstruction of parietal lymphatic drainage. Malignant effusions are mostly exudative (90%), often with a very high LDH, low pH and low glucose. Cytology of the pleural fluid has a high diagnostic yield. Symptomatic pleural effusions may respond to therapy for the underlying malignancy, although palliative obliteration of the pleural space (**pleurodesis**) is often necessary to relieve dyspnoea or chest pain.

Mesothelioma is an uncommon malignancy that originates in the pleura and/or peritoneum. Over 75% of cases develop 20–30 years after occupational asbestos exposure. Asbestos may also cause benign pleural effusions or calcified plaques on the parietal pleura in the lower lungs or along the diaphragmatic surface. Mesothelioma typically develops in men aged 50–70, presenting with insidious dyspnoea and aching chest pain. Chest X-rays usually show unilateral pleural effusion (Fig. 28b), and computed tomography (CT) shows fibrotic encasement of the pleural space. Pleural fluid cytology is not usually diagnostic. Thoracoscopic biopsies have the highest yield. Treatment is generally palliative, including pleurodesis. The prognosis is poor, with a median survival of approximately 1 year.

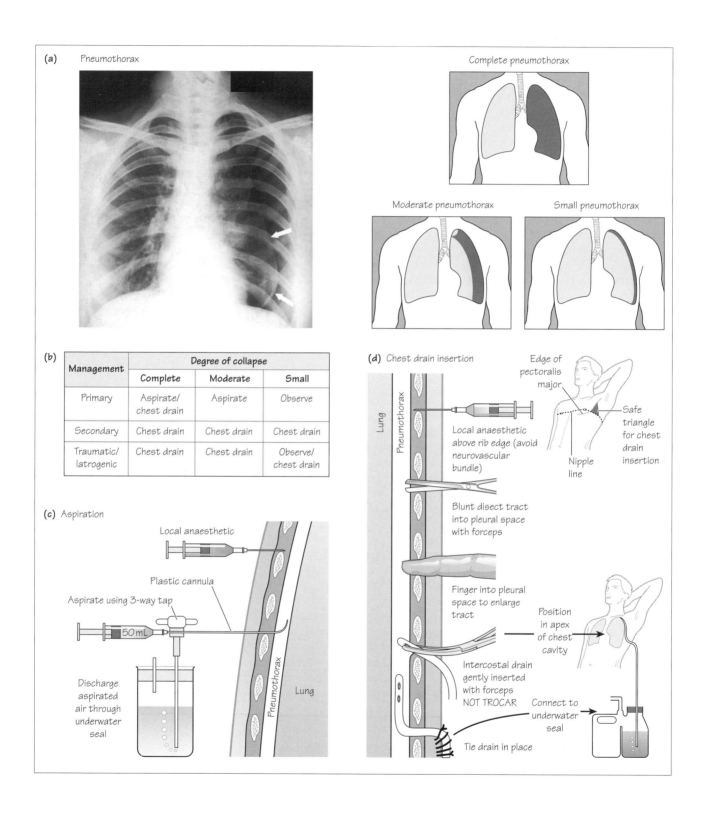

(a) Pneumothorax

Complete pneumothorax

Moderate pneumothorax

Small pneumothorax

(b)

Management	Degree of collapse		
	Complete	Moderate	Small
Primary	Aspirate/ chest drain	Aspirate	Observe
Secondary	Chest drain	Chest drain	Chest drain
Traumatic/ Iatrogenic	Chest drain	Chest drain	Observe/ chest drain

(c) Aspiration

Local anaesthetic

Plastic cannula

Aspirate using 3-way tap

50 mL

Discharge aspirated air through underwater seal

Pneumothorax

Lung

(d) Chest drain insertion

Lung

Pneumothorax

Local anaesthetic above rib edge (avoid neurovascular bundle)

Blunt disect tract into pleural space with forceps

Finger into pleural space to enlarge tract

Intercostal drain gently inserted with forceps NOT TROCAR

Tie drain in place

Edge of pectoralis major

Safe triangle for chest drain insertion

Nipple line

Position in apex of chest cavity

Connect to underwater seal

Definition

Pneumothorax is a collection of air between the visceral and parietal pleura, causing a real rather than potential pleural space (Fig. 29a).

Causes, epidemiology and prognosis

Pneumothorax may be categorized into the following types.

Primary spontaneous pneumothorax (PSP): characteristically affects tall, narrow-chested, young (20–40-year-old), male (M:F 5:1) adults. It is the commonest type of pneumothorax (prevalence 8/100 000/year, rising to 200/100 000/year in subjects >1.9 m in height). There is usually no antecedent history of chest disease, and underlying lung disease is unlikely. It occurs following rupture of small apical subpleural air cysts ('blebs'). Often the pneumothorax is small and in some cases it can be managed without drainage or with simple aspiration (see below) on an outpatient basis. Ipsilateral recurrence is common; after a second and third pneumothorax, recurrence rates are 60% and 80%, respectively. **Pleurodesis** (fusion of the visceral and parietal pleural) by medical (pleural insertion of bleomycin or talc) or surgical (abrasion of the pleural lining) means is recommended after the second pneumothorax (or first, if the risk of a second pneumothorax would be high as in a mountain climber). It is usually curative.

Secondary pneumothorax is associated with respiratory disease, most commonly **obstructive** (COPD, asthma), **fibrotic** (cryptogenic fibrosing alveolitis, CFA) or **infective** (tuberculosis, pneumonia) and occasionally rare or inherited disorders (**lymphangioleiomyomatosis, Marfan's, cystic fibrosis**) that disrupt lung architecture. Secondary pneumothorax is more serious than PSP, because the patient has less respiratory reserve to deal with the lung collapse due to underlying lung disease. These patients require admission to hospital and even a small pneumothorax will need **intercostal tube drainage** (Fig. 29b).

Traumatic/iatrogenic pneumothorax: often follows blunt (road traffic accidents) or penetrating (fractured ribs, stab wounds) chest trauma. Intensive-care unit patients with lung disease are at particular risk of pneumothorax due to the high pressures (**barotrauma**) and alveolar overdistension ('**volutrauma**') associated with mechanical ventilation. 'Protective' ventilation strategies using low-pressure, low-volume ventilation reduce this risk. Therapeutic procedures (line insertion, chest wall surgery, pleural biopsy) are the commonest iatrogenic causes of pneumothorax.

A **tension pneumothorax** may complicate primary, secondary or traumatic pneumothoraces, but is most common during **mechanical ventilation** and following **trauma**. It occurs when air accumulates in the pleural cavity faster than it can be removed. The increase in intrathoracic pressure causes mediastinal shift, compression of functioning lung, inhibition of venous return and shock due to reduced cardiac output. It is a **medical emergency** and fatal if not rapidly relieved by drainage. Detection is a clinical diagnosis; awaiting chest X-ray (CXR) confirmation may be life-threatening. Immediate drainage with a 14-G needle in the second intercostal space in the midclavicular is essential. A characteristic 'hiss' of escaping gas confirms the diagnosis. A chest drain is then inserted (Fig. 29b).

Clinical evaluation

A pneumothorax should be considered in any patient who suddenly becomes breathless for no obvious reason, particularly if there is underlying lung disease. Sudden onset of **sharp pleuritic pain** and **breathlessness** are the commonest presenting symptoms. Most primary spontaneous pneumothoraces are small, defined as occupying less than 30% of the diameter of the hemithorax (Fig. 29b), and cause few symptoms other than pain. Clinical signs can be surprisingly difficult to detect, but in larger pneumothoraxes reduced air entry and hyperresonant percussion over one hemithorax are characteristic and may be associated with tachypnoea and cyanosis. Occasionally, air may track into the mediastinum (pneumomediastinum), into the subcutaneous tissue at the root of the neck or along the tract of a chest drain, causing subcutaneous emphysema. Subcutaneous emphysema can cause extensive facial and body swelling and has a characteristic cracking sensation on palpation. It usually subsides without complications following adequate drainage of the pneumothorax.

Investigation

Routine monitoring procedures may detect tachycardia, hypotension and desaturation at the onset of a pneumothorax. Routine blood tests are normal, although blood gases demonstrate hypoxaemia and hypocapnia. A chest radiograph in inspiration will confirm the diagnosis. Localized pneumothoraxes following trauma or mechanical ventilation may only be visible on a chest computed tomography (CT) scan. Other investigations are only of value in determining the nature of underlying lung disease.

Management

Immediate supportive therapy includes supplemental oxygen by face-mask and analgesia. Treatment of a pneumothorax is dependent on the cause, size and symptoms and is summarized in Fig. 29b. A tension pneumothorax must be drained immediately (see above). A small PSP (<30%) may be managed without drainage on an outpatient basis. Follow-up radiography will confirm gradual reabsorption of pleural air. Moderate (>30%) and even large PSP, with significant symptoms, may be successfully aspirated. Following infiltration of local anaesthetic, a 16-G cannula is inserted into the second intercostal space in the midclavicular line. The needle is withdrawn and air is aspirated through the cannula using a 50-mL syringe and a three-way tap connected to an underwater seal (Fig. 29c). Aspiration is discontinued when resistance is felt, if excessive coughing occurs or if more than 2.5 L have been aspirated. Successful aspiration is confirmed on a repeat chest radiograph. Following aspiration, all patients should be admitted overnight. Intercostal chest drainage (Fig. 29d) may be required for moderate or large PSP with hypoxaemic respiratory failure or if aspiration is unsuccessful. In general, all secondary and traumatic pneumothoraces will require admission to hospital and a chest drain. Suction (5–50 cmH$_2$O) should be applied using a high-flow system (i.e. 'wall' suction) if a persistent leak develops. The correct pressure is that which opposes the visceral and parietal pleura, allowing pleurodesis. Early thoracic surgical advice should be obtained if the pleural surfaces cannot be opposed, as this suggests development of a bronchopleural fistula, which may require surgical correction.

30 Cystic fibrosis and bronchiectasis

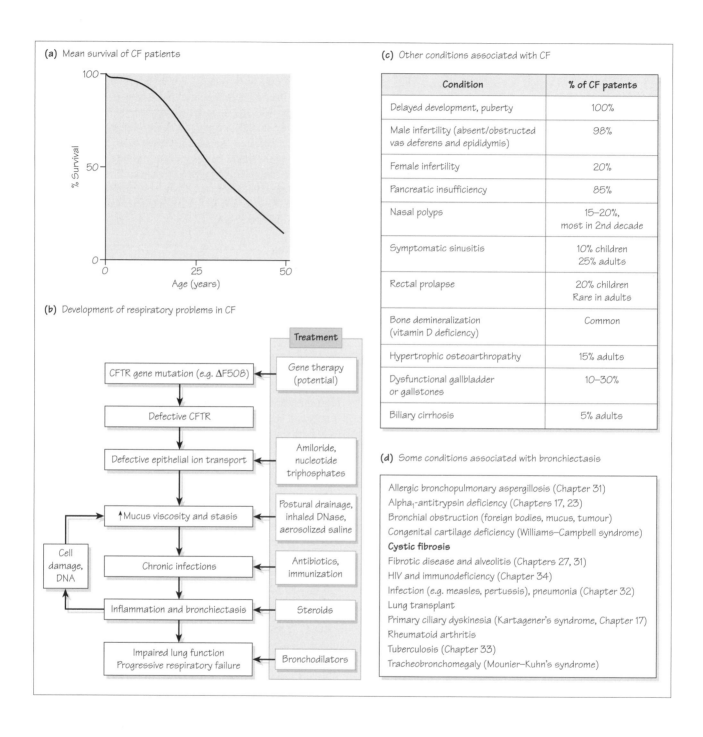

(a) Mean survival of CF patients

y-axis: % Survival (0, 50, 100)
x-axis: Age (years) (0, 25, 50)

(b) Development of respiratory problems in CF

Treatment

Pathway	Treatment
CFTR gene mutation (e.g. ΔF508)	Gene therapy (potential)
Defective CFTR	
Defective epithelial ion transport	Amiloride, nucleotide triphosphates
↑Mucus viscosity and stasis	Postural drainage, inhaled DNase, aerosolized saline
Chronic infections	Antibiotics, immunization
Inflammation and bronchiectasis	Steroids
Impaired lung function Progressive respiratory failure	Bronchodilators

Cell damage, DNA

(c) Other conditions associated with CF

Condition	% of CF patents
Delayed development, puberty	100%
Male infertility (absent/obstructed vas deferens and epididymis)	98%
Female infertility	20%
Pancreatic insufficiency	85%
Nasal polyps	15–20%, most in 2nd decade
Symptomatic sinusitis	10% children 25% adults
Rectal prolapse	20% children Rare in adults
Bone demineralization (vitamin D deficiency)	Common
Hypertrophic osteoarthropathy	15% adults
Dysfunctional gallbladder or gallstones	10–30%
Biliary cirrhosis	5% adults

(d) Some conditions associated with bronchiectasis

Allergic bronchopulmonary aspergillosis (Chapter 31)
Alpha₁-antitrypsin deficiency (Chapters 17, 23)
Bronchial obstruction (foreign bodies, mucus, tumour)
Congenital cartilage deficiency (Williams–Campbell syndrome)
Cystic fibrosis
Fibrotic disease and alveolitis (Chapters 27, 31)
HIV and immunodeficiency (Chapter 34)
Infection (e.g. measles, pertussis), pneumonia (Chapter 32)
Lung transplant
Primary ciliary dyskinesia (Kartagener's syndrome, Chapter 17)
Rheumatoid arthritis
Tuberculosis (Chapter 33)
Tracheobronchomegaly (Mounier–Kuhn's syndrome)

Cystic fibrosis (CF) is the primary cause of severe chronic lung disease in children, although 90% of children now survive into their second decade (Fig. 30a). CF is characterized by **chronic bronchopulmonary infection** and airway obstruction (Fig. 30b) and by **exocrine pancreatic insufficiency** with consequent effects on gut function, nutrition and development. The key feature of CF is **increased viscosity** and **subsequent stasis of epithelial mucus.**

There is usually an **increased salt content of sweat.** Figure 30c shows some associated disorders.

CF is an **autosomal recessive trait** that is the most common genetic cause of morbidity and mortality in the white population, with a prevalence of around one in 2000 live births; nearly 5% of whites of European descent are heterozygous carriers. Prevalence is far less in others, being ~1 in 17 000 for those of African descent. CF is due to mutations in a gene on chromosome 7 encoding for the **cystic fibrosis transmembrane conductance regulator** (CFTR), a cyclic adenosine monophosphate (cAMP)-regulated epithelial chloride channel that can also alter activity of other ionic transporters. Dysfunction of CFTR impairs epithelial chloride, sodium and water transfer and thus causes **reduced mucus hydration** and **increased viscosity** (Chapter 17). Over 800 mutations in the CFTR gene have been described, but the most common, found in ~65% of patients with CF, is deletion of the phenylalanine codon at position 508, the **ΔF508** mutation.

Clinical features

The lungs of neonates with CF are often normal, but rapid development of respiratory symptoms, including refractory cough and infections, is usual. CF patients nearly always have an increased lung volume and **finger clubbing** (increased curvature of the nail and loss of normal angle between nail and nail bed). Recurrent bronchopulmonary infections, primarily as a result of defective mucus clearance, are rarely cleared once established and eventually result in **bronchiectasis** (see below), extensive lung damage and dysfunction. Spontaneous **pneumothorax** (Chapter 29) and **haemoptysis** (spitting blood; see Chapter 40) are not uncommon. About 10% of neonates present with meconium ileus (failure to pass meconium), which can cause death in the first days of life; 20% of older patients exhibit a similar ileal obstruction (**meconium ileus equivalent**, MIE). Eighty-five per cent of patients have steatorrhoea (high fat stools) as a result of pancreatic insufficiency. Some patients have only mild respiratory symptoms for many years, but this is inevitably followed by a characteristic increase in the frequency and severity of periods of exacerbation of symptoms (cough, dyspnoea, loss of appetite). Eventually, severe restrictions in activity herald the end-stage disease, followed by respiratory failure, hypoxaemia, pulmonary hypertension and death.

Diagnosis

Several factors need to be taken into account, including a **family history** of the disease and the presence of typical respiratory and gastrointestinal disorders (Fig. 30c). A **sweat chloride or sodium** concentration above 60 mmol/L is diagnostic when coupled with such disorders, although ~1% of CF patients may have normal sweat electrolytes. DNA analysis can detect known mutations (e.g. ΔF508), but is limited by the high number of unknown mutations. In later disease chest X-rays can detect bronchiectasis (see below). Neonates can be screened for CF by blood immunoreactive trypsin, which may detect many, but not all cases.

Management

The primary objectives of treatment are to **control infection, promote mucus clearance** and **improve nutrition**. Early antibiotic therapy is crucial to inhibit progression of the disease. Choice of antibiotic is determined following identification of infecting organisms. The dose should be higher in CF patients and the course longer. Development of resistance is a key problem and is transferable; segregation of patients is thus advisable. Adequate immunization for measles, pertussis and influenza is important, as these organisms are particularly dangerous in CF.

Clearance: training by physiotherapists in postural drainage (tipping the body so that the infected lobe is uppermost) is vital, coupled with chest percussion to mobilize secretions to the upper airways where they can be coughed up. Such treatment is prescribed one to four times a day. Recently introduced therapies include inhalation of DNase, an enzyme that breaks down DNA from dead cells which contributes to mucus viscosity. Inhalation of aerosolized saline may improve mucus hydration, as may blockade of sodium reabsorption with amiloride or stimulation of chloride secretion with nucleotide triphosphates. Cough should never be suppressed, as it is an important method of clearance.

Other therapies: bronchodilators (β-agonists) may improve lung function and corticosteroids may assist inflammation in some patients. A potential therapy under intense investigation is gene transfer of the normal CFTR gene. In end-stage respiratory disease a lung transplant should be considered.

Nutrition: most patients with CF require pancreatic enzymes with meals, supplemented with vitamins. High-calorific foods should be advised.

Bronchiectasis

Bronchiectasis is an abnormal and permanent dilation of proximal (>2 mm) bronchi due to inflammation and subsequent destruction of the elastic and muscular components of their walls (see also Chapter 40). It is normally associated with defects in **mucociliary clearance** (Chapter 17) and **persistent respiratory infections**. Onset is often in childhood, following pulmonary infections complicating measles or pertussis. Since the introduction of antibiotics, the most common cause of bronchiectasis is now CF (Fig. 30d), except in poorly resourced countries. Symptoms depend on the severity and location of diseased bronchi, but commonly include persistent productive cough, with large quantities of foul-smelling purulent sputum as the disease worsens. Severity has been correlated with the volume of sputum produced, but not with dyspnoea. Haemoptysis and recurrent pneumonia or abscesses are common; haemoptysis is normally mild, but can become life-threatening, particularly in CF patients. Fever, anaemia and weight loss may accompany the disease. Patients often develop finger clubbing, metastatic abscesses, respiratory failure and amyloidosis. Chest X-rays and high-resolution computed tomography (HRCT) can often detect the dilated and thickened bronchi (Chapter 40). **Management** is similar to that for CF, though without the nutritional requirements.

31 Occupational and environmental-related lung disease

(a) Common examples of irritant gases and other agents causing lung-specific responses

Agent	Source	Response
Ammonia	Industrial refrigeration leaks, fertilizers	**Low exposure**
Chlorine gas	Industrial leakage, water purification including swimming pools, household bleach (liquid/powder) interactions	Exacerbations of asthma and COPD Enhanced response to allergen
Hydrogen sulphide	Sewers and manure pits, fossil fuel extraction	**Moderate exposure** Mild mucosal irritation Airway inflammation and bronchiolitis
Nitrogen dioxide Nitrogen oxides	Vehicle exhausts, welding, power stations, oil refineries, gas and oil burning equipment, organic decomposition, structural or polymer fibres	**Severe exposure** Epithelial damage leading to diffuse alveolar damage Pulmonary oedema and ARDS
Ozone	Vehicle exhausts, welding, copiers, ozone generators, bleaching, water treatment, plasma welding	**In some cases – late response (2–8 weeks)** Bronchiolitis obliterans after initial recovery
Sulphur dioxide	Combustion of fossil fuels, power stations, oil refineries, smelters, oil burning heaters, mining, ore refining, cement manufacturing, refrigeration plants	**Also**: direct bronchoconstriction, especially in asthmatics
Acrolein, aldehydes	Structural or wildland fires, other combustion	**Also**: strongly pro-inflammatory (esp. acrolein)
Diesel particulates (<10μm)	Diesel engines	Airway/alveolar inflammation Increased deaths in elderly
Heavy metals (cadmium, mercury)	Welding, brazing, metal cutting, metal reclamation	Acute pneumonitis 12–24 hours after exposure
Paraquat	Ingestion of herbicides	Accelerated, chemically induced pulmonary fibrosis
Polycyclic hydrocarbons Hydrocarbons	Diesel exhaust, tobacco smoke Ingestion of hydrocarbons (children)	Cancer Aspiration hydrocarbon pneumonitis

(b) Typical causes of allergic alveolitis

Disease/occupation	Material	Causative agent
Farmer's lung	Mouldy hay or other vegetable matter	Thermophilic actinomycetes bacteria (*Saccharopolyspora rectivirgula*, *Thermoactinomyces* species)
Bagassosis	Sugar cane	
Mushroom workers	Compost	
Humidifier fever	Contaminated water	– Also *Klebsiella oxytoca*, amoebae
Pigeon fancier's (breeder's) lung	Feathers and excreta	Avian proteins
Farmers, sawmill, tobacco, esparto grass and brewery workers	Fungal contamination of materials	Primarily *Aspergillus* species
Cheese, laboratory, cork workers	Fungal contamination of materials	Primarily *Penicillium* species
Household	Fungal infestations of damp walls and woodwork	Multiple fungal species
– other bacterial causes	Contamination of water, wood shavings etc.	*Bacillus subtilis*, *Klebsiella*, *Epicoccum nigrum*, non-tubercular mycobacteria

The most common form of occupational and environmental lung disease is **asthma** (Chapters 21 and 22). See Chapter 36 for lung cancer.

Response to acute lung irritants

Inhaled irritants (Fig. 31a) cause exacerbation of asthma and chronic obstructive pulmonary disease (COPD), coughing and dyspnoea through activation of irritant receptors (Chapter 11), and irritation of mucus membranes. Highly soluble agents (e.g. ammonia, sulphur dioxide) cause immediate irritation in the upper airways, whereas less soluble agents (e.g. chlorine, ozone) favour deeper penetration to alveolar epithelial cells, which are particularly susceptible to injury. High concentrations lead to extensive lung injury, primarily by damage to epithelium, consequent inflammation and **pulmonary oedema**. Development of **acute respiratory distress syndrome** (ARDS) is common, and treatment is similar (Chapter 35). Some patients who initially recover from moderate or severe exposure may subsequently develop **bronchiolitis obliterans** (obliteration of bronchioles by fibrous growth) after 2–8 weeks. Although steroids may slow progression, prognosis is often poor.

Inhalation of mineral dusts (pneumoconiosis)

Coal workers' pneumoconiosis (CWP) is caused by inhalation of coal or carbon dust. In **simple CWP**, the upper lobes of the lung contain small (<4 mm), round opacities (coal macules) consisting of dust, dust-laden macrophages and fibroblasts. These may enlarge to coal nodules, which are fibrosed. Weakening of bronchiolar walls leads to focal emphysema, which together with macules is characteristic of CWP. Simple CWP is often described as symptomless, with no discernible change in lung function. It can, however, develop into progressive massive fibrosis (PMF), with black fibrotic masses from 1 cm to several centimeters in diameter that may have necrotic cavities. Obliteration and disruption of airways results in emphysema. Patients show irreversible airflow limitation, loss of lung volume and elastic recoil, and reduced $D_L\text{co}$, with significant breathlessness on exertion. Treatment is limited, and similar to other progressive fibrotic diseases (Chapter 27). **Caplan's syndrome** is a nodular form of CWP associated with the defective immunology of rheumatoid disease; it may also occur with asbestosis or silicosis.

Asbestos is a fibrous mixture of silicates that is highly resistant to degradation. The fibres are 1–2 μm wide, but up to 50 μm (**blue asbestos**; crocidolite) or 2 cm (**white asbestos**; chrysotile) long. They are thus easily trapped in the lung. Blue asbestos is far more dangerous. Regulations have reduced exposure since the 1980s, but the presence of asbestos in buildings and the long interval between exposure and disease development mean that asbestos-related disease will be encountered for some time. **Asbestos bodies** (protein-covered fibres) in the lungs are indicative of exposure, but not disease. The type and extent of disease largely depend on exposure. **Asbestosis** is a fibrous lung disease developing up to 10 years after heavy exposure. Patients present with progressive dyspnoea, basal crackles on inspiration, and sometimes finger clubbing. There is a restrictive lung function defect and reduced $D_L\text{co}$, with diffuse streaky shadows on X-ray and thickening of visceral pleura; honeycomb lung is often prominent in the lower lobes. Prognosis is poor.

Mesothelioma (Chapter 28) can develop up to 40 years after light exposure, and is invariably fatal. Milder forms of asbestos-induced pleural disease produce dyspnoea and restrictive defects coupled with pleural thickening, pleural plaques (distinctive partially calcified lesions generally on parietal pleura) or effusions, with scattered fibrotic foci. No treatment is effective for asbestos-related disease, as the stimulus remains in the lungs. Asbestos-related lung cancer is discussed in Chapter 36.

Silicosis is a fibrotic disease caused by inhalation of silica. Occupations at risk include mining, quarrying, stoneworking, manufacture of abrasives, foundry work and glassworking. Its prevalence in developed nations is low. Silica is very toxic to macrophages and thus highly fibrogenic. Chronic silicosis (over decades) is characterized by **silicotic nodules** of collagen around a cell-free core, first developing in hilar lymph nodes. In acute silicosis due to heavy exposure, severe dyspnoea may develop over months. The clinical features of silicosis are similar to PMF.

Berylliosis is caused by systemic poisoning by inhaled beryllium (electronics, high tensile alloys), giving rise to symptoms similar to sarcoidosis (Chapter 28). Industrial regulations have made this a rarity.

Inhalation of organic material

Extrinsic allergic alveolitis (or **hypersensitivity pneumonitis**) is a diffuse inflammatory disease of small airways and alveoli caused by allergens, primarily microbial spores, that are small enough to reach the alveoli (Fig. 31b). The most common example is **farmer's lung**, caused by dust from mouldy hay or plants contaminated with **thermophilic actinomycetes** bacteria, which thrive in warm moist conditions. Typically, symptoms occur several hours after exposure, and include fever, dyspnoea and cough. Although early removal of antigen exposure results in rapid recovery, continuous exposure leads to progressive **interstitial fibrosis** (Chapter 27), with infiltration of inflammatory cells and formation of **granulomas** (chronically inflamed tissue masses characterized by multinucleate giant cells). Patients present with dyspnoea, restrictive defects and decreased $D_L\text{co}$. Fluffy nodular shadowing or ground glass opacity may be shown in X-ray, with honeycomb lung (Chapter 27) in severe cases. Detailed histories are required to establish antigens, with confirmation by precipitating antibodies in serum. Bronchiolar lavage or even lung biopsy may be required where diagnosis is not clear. **Management** centres on abolishing antigen exposure. High-dose oral corticosteroids can regress early disease, but established disease with fibrosis is irreversible and can progress to respiratory failure. **Differential diagnosis** includes asthma (Chapter 21), sarcoidosis (Chapter 27), viral and mycoplasma pneumonias (Chapter 32) and mycobacterial infections.

Byssinosis occurs in workers handling raw cotton, flax and hemp. It is characterized by chest tightness, cough and/or shortness of breath on the first day back at work, with recovery as the week progresses. It is primarily due to acute bronchoconstriction, possibly related to contaminating bacterial endotoxins; byssinosis is not induced by processed cotton or linen (flax). Long-term exposure causes a disease similar to chronic bronchitis (Chapter 23), with chronic productive cough, progressive decline in lung function and disability.

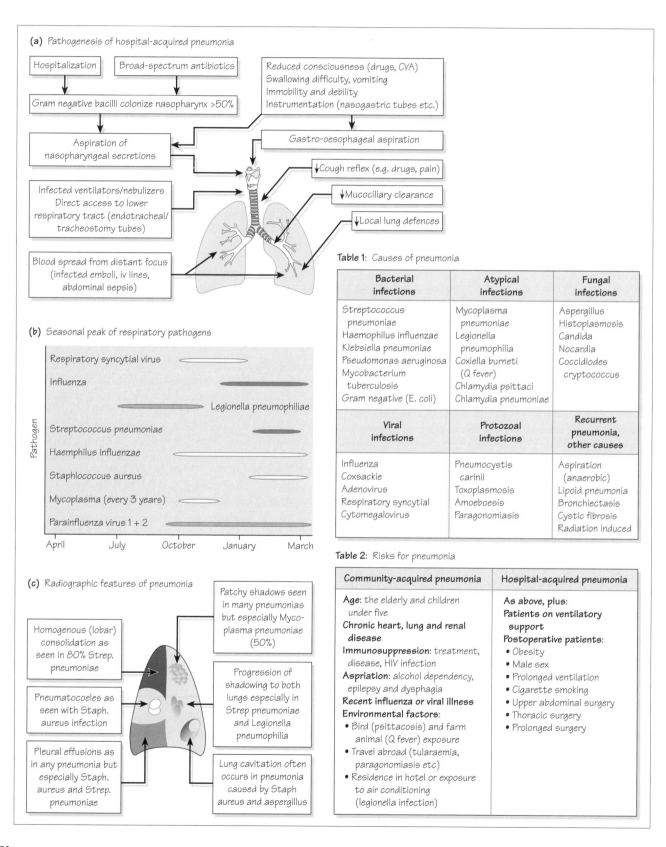

(a) Pathogenesis of hospital-acquired pneumonia

Hospitalization → Gram negative bacilli colonize nasopharynx >50%

Broad-spectrum antibiotics → Gram negative bacilli colonize nasopharynx >50%

Reduced consciousness (drugs, CVA)
Swallowing difficulty, vomiting
Immobility and debility
Instrumentation (nasogastric tubes etc.)

Gram negative bacilli colonize nasopharynx >50%

Aspiration of nasopharyngeal secretions

Gastro-oesophageal aspiration

↓Cough reflex (e.g. drugs, pain)

Infected ventilators/nebulizers
Direct access to lower respiratory tract (endotracheal/ tracheostomy tubes)

↓Mucociliary clearance

↓Local lung defences

Blood spread from distant focus (infected emboli, iv lines, abdominal sepsis)

(b) Seasonal peak of respiratory pathogens

Pathogen:
Respiratory syncytial virus
Influenza
Legionella pneumophiliae
Streptococcus pneumoniae
Haemphilus influenzae
Staphlococcus aureus
Mycoplasma (every 3 years)
Parainfluenza virus 1 + 2

April — July — October — January — March

(c) Radiographic features of pneumonia

Patchy shadows seen in many pneumonias but especially Myco-plasma pneumoniae (50%)

Homogenous (lobar) consolidation as seen in 80% Strep. pneumoniae

Pneumatocoeles as seen with Staph. aureus infection

Progression of shadowing to both lungs especially in Strep pneumoniae and Legionella pneumophilia

Pleural effusions as in any pneumonia but especially Staph. aureus and Strep. pneumoniae

Lung cavitation often occurs in pneumonia caused by Staph aureus and aspergillus

Table 1: Causes of pneumonia

Bacterial infections	Atypical infections	Fungal infections
Streptococcus pneumoniae	Mycoplasma pneumoniae	Aspergillus
Haemophilus influenzae	Legionella pneumophilia	Histoplasmosis
Klebsiella pneumoniae	Coxiella burneti (Q fever)	Candida
Pseudomonas aeruginosa	Chlamydia psittaci	Nocardia
Mycobacterium tuberculosis	Chlamydia pneumoniae	Coccidiodes cryptococcus
Gram negative (E. coli)		

Viral infections	Protozoal infections	Recurrent pneumonia, other causes
Influenza	Pneumocystis carinii	Aspiration (anaerobic)
Coxsackie	Toxoplasmosis	Lipoid pneumonia
Adenovirus	Amoeboesis	Bronchiectasis
Respiratory syncytial	Paragonomiasis	Cystic fibrosis
Cytomegalovirus		Radiation induced

Table 2: Risks for pneumonia

Community-acquired pneumonia	Hospital-acquired pneumonia
Age: the elderly and children under five	**As above, plus:**
Chronic heart, lung and renal disease	**Patients on ventilatory support**
Immunosuppression: treatment, disease, HIV infection	**Postoperative patients:**
Aspriation: alcohol dependency, epilepsy and dysphagia	• Obesity
Recent influenza or viral illness	• Male sex
Environmental factors:	• Prolonged ventilation
• Bird (psittacosis) and farm animal (Q fever) exposure	• Cigarette smoking
• Travel abroad (tularaemia, paragonomiasis etc)	• Upper abdominal surgery
• Residence in hotel or exposure to air conditioning (legionella infection)	• Thoracic surgery
	• Prolonged surgery

Pneumonia is defined as an acute lower respiratory tract illness, usually due to infection, associated with fever, focal chest symptoms (signs) and recently developed shadowing on CXR. It is caused by a wide variety of microorganisms and pathological insults, some of which are shown in Table 1.

Classification

Classification of pneumonia by **radiographic appearance** (lobar pneumonia or bronchopneumonia) gives little practical information about cause or appropriate treatment. Classification by microbiological pathogen (streptococcal, viral, fungal) most accurately defines the course, clinical picture and outcome, but is not practical in the clinical situation where microbiological diagnosis is often delayed. The following classification scheme is widely accepted:

1 Community-acquired pneumonia is common, and one in 1000 of the population require admission for pneumonia each year. The most likely pathogens in these cases are *Streptococcus pneumoniae* (60–75%), *Mycoplasma pneumoniae* (5–18%), *influenza A* (7–8%), *Haemophilus influenza* (4–5%) and *Legionella* (2–5%). Mortality is ~5–18% of admissions.

2 Hospital-acquired (nosocomial) pneumonia is any lower respiratory tract infection developing two or more days after hospital admission and not apparent at admission. Pneumonia is the 3rd commonest nosocomial infection after wound and urinary tract infections, and occurs in ~4 per 1000 hospital patients; its pathogenesis is outlined in Fig. 32a. Likely pathogens are **Gram-negative bacilli** (65–70%) including *Klebsiella, Pseudomonas, Escherichia coli, Proteus* and **Staphylococcus** (10–15%). Mortality is ~20–30% (50% with bacteraemia).

3 Other pneumonias include **aspiration and anaerobic** pneumonia, pneumonia in the **immunocompromised** patient (e.g. *Pneumocystis carinii* in human immunodeficiency virus (HIV) patients, Chapter 34) and **recurrent pneumonia** due to cystic fibrosis or bronchiectasis (Chapter 30).

Risks

Common risk factors are shown in Table 2, and are affected by **season and locality**. Pneumonia is more common in winter due to increased incidence of viral infections (*influenza, respiratory syncytial virus*); seasonal peaks of common respiratory pathogens are shown in Fig. 32b. Variations may occur due to 3-yearly epidemics of *Mycoplasma pneumoniae* and irregular epidemics of *influenza*. Epidemics of *Legionella pneumophila* (Legionnaires disease) and *Coxiella burnetii* (Q fever) are usually localized.

Diagnosis

General features include malaise, fever, rigors, myalgia, cyanosis, tachycardia and a respiratory rate >20/min. **Specific symptoms** include dyspnoea, pleuritic chest pain, cough, wheeze and sputum production, with **focal signs** of dullness, crepitations, bronchial breathing and pleuritic rub. In the very young or old and those with **atypical pneumonia** (*Mycoplasma, Legionella,* psittacosis), non-respiratory features may predominate (headache, confusion, diarrhoea, rash, cyanosis).

Severity should be assessed. In community-acquired pneumonia, the following features are associated with increased mortality, and indicate the need for transfer to a critical care unit:

Clinical: age >60 years, respiratory rate >30/min, diastolic blood pressure <60 mmHg, new atrial fibrillation, confusion.
Laboratory: raised serum urea >7 mmol/L, serum albumin <35 g/L, hypoxaemia ($PO_2 < 8$ kPa), leucopenia (white cell count $<4 \times 10^9/L$), leucocytosis ($>20 \times 10^9/L$), multilobar involvement and bacteraemia.

Complications of pneumonia include pleural effusion/empyema (Chapter 28), lung abscess, respiratory failure (Chapter 20), bacteraemia and meningitis, and rarely pericarditis, myocarditis or cholestatic jaundice.

Investigations: early identification of likely pathogens aids management, although no microorganism is isolated in 33–50% of patients, due to previous antibiotic therapy or inadequate specimens. Chest X-rays (Fig. 32c) and CT scans aid diagnosis and detect complications. **Routine blood tests:** white cell count ($>15 \times 10^9/L$ = pneumonia, $<3 \times 10^9/L$ = poor prognosis), haemolysis and cold agglutinins may indicate mycoplasma infection. **Liver function tests** may indicate *Legionella* or *Mycoplasma* infection. **Blood gases** identify respiratory failure. **Blood cultures, sputum for acid-fast bacillus (AFB), Gram stain, culture** and **sensitivity** identify the pathogen. **Serology** detects *Legionella* and *Mycoplasma* pneumonia. **Bronchoscopy** provides specimens for microbiology. **Pneumococcal antigen detection** (serum, urine) and **urine enzyme-linked immunoassay (ELISA)** for *Legionella* infection are occasionally useful.

Management

Supportive measures include O_2 by face mask to maintain $P_aO_2 > 8$ kPa or O_2 saturation > 90%, and intravenous fluids and inotropic drugs may be required for haemodynamic stability. **Ventilatory support:** continuous positive airway pressure (CPAP), non-invasive positive pressure ventilation (NIPPV), or mechanical ventilation may be required with respiratory failure (Chapters 20 and 38).

Antibiotic therapy: as microbiological results may not be available for 24 h, antibiotic therapy is initially given 'blind'; appropriate therapy depends on how the pneumonia presents, and must be amended as soon as the microbiological results and antibiotic sensitivities become available.

Community-acquired pneumonia: In the hospitalized patient, antibiotic therapy must cover streptococcal pneumonia and atypical pneumonias (*Mycoplasma, Legionella*). **Erythromycin** with or without **cefuroxime** is recommended. Staphylococcal infection is common after influenza, and *Haemophilus influenzae* is associated with chronic lung disease.

Hospital-acquired pneumonia: antibiotic therapy for Gram-negative bacilli and staphylococci is required. Broad-spectrum antibiotics, including combinations of **cephalosporins, quinolones, gentamicin** and **antistaphylococcal** drugs, are recommended.

Aspiration pneumonia: anaerobes must be covered in addition to other microbes (add **metronidazole**).

Pneumonia in the immunocompromised: broad-spectrum antibiotics are required after chemotherapy. HIV-infected patients may require specific therapy for viral (cytomegalovirus) and protozoal infections; *Pneumocystis carinii* pneumonia is treated with **steroids** and high-dose co-trimoxazole (**Septrin**).

33 Pulmonary tuberculosis

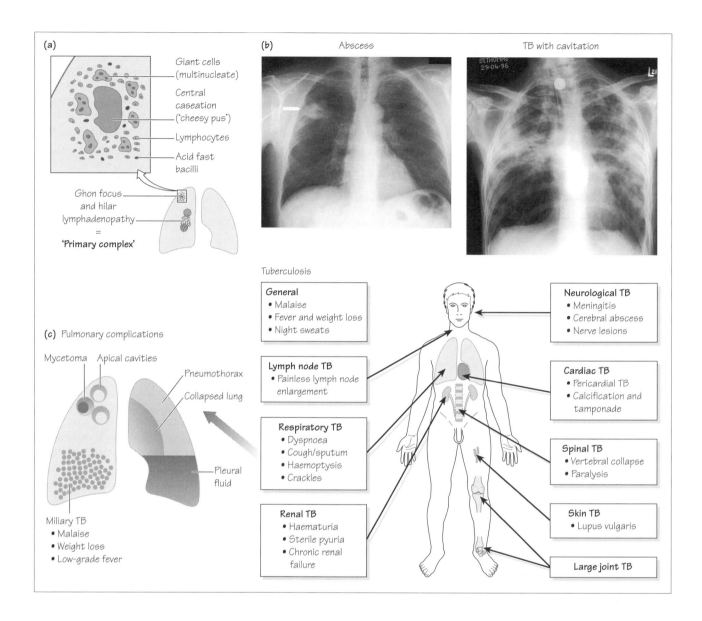

(a)

Giant cells (multinucleate)

Central caseation ('cheesy pus')

Lymphocytes

Acid fast bacilli

Ghon focus and hilar lymphadenopathy
=
'Primary complex'

(b) Abscess

TB with cavitation

(c) Pulmonary complications

Mycetoma   Apical cavities

Pneumothorax

Collapsed lung

Pleural fluid

Miliary TB
• Malaise
• Weight loss
• Low-grade fever

Tuberculosis

General
• Malaise
• Fever and weight loss
• Night sweats

Lymph node TB
• Painless lymph node enlargement

Respiratory TB
• Dyspnoea
• Cough/sputum
• Haemoptysis
• Crackles

Renal TB
• Haematuria
• Sterile pyuria
• Chronic renal failure

Neurological TB
• Meningitis
• Cerebral abscess
• Nerve lesions

Cardiac TB
• Pericardial TB
• Calcification and tamponade

Spinal TB
• Vertebral collapse
• Paralysis

Skin TB
• Lupus vulgaris

Large joint TB

Epidemiology and aetiology

Worldwide, tuberculosis (TB) affects 10 million people and causes 3 million deaths each year. In developed countries, it is an uncommon disease affecting approximately one per 10 000 population. Pulmonary tuberculosis is most common in Asian, Chinese and West Indian people. Airborne transmission and close contact with an infected person spread the disease. Those who are elderly, malnourished or immunosuppressed (HIV infection, diabetes mellitus, corticosteroid therapy, alcoholism, intercurrent lymphoma) are more susceptible. Improved housing and nutrition reduce the incidence of tuberculosis.

Pathogenesis

Primary pulmonary tuberculosis is caused by the acid-fast bacil-lus, *Mycobacterium tuberculosis*. The inhaled bacillus infects well-ventilated, poorly perfused upper lung lobes subpleurally. A **granuloma** forms (Fig. 33a) known as the **Ghon focus**, and with the enlarged hilar lymph nodes draining the affected lung is known as the '**primary complex**' (Fig. 33a). This process occurs over 3–8 weeks, and is accompanied by the development of an inflammatory reaction to the injection of tubercular protein (**tuberculin**) into the skin, which can be used as a diagnostic test (**Heaf** or **Mantoux** test). Complete healing usually follows, with fibrosis and calcification of the Ghon focus and immunity to further infection.

Post-primary pulmonary tuberculosis occurs if the Ghon focus fails to heal due to poor host defences, or following reactivation at a later date. It is potentially fatal. Local dissemination causes **tuberculous pneumonia** and **pleural effusions**. Blood-borne spread may affect the meninges or individual organs. In a few cases, widespread infection involves many tissues and is known as **miliary tuberculosis**.

Clinical features

Primary pulmonary tuberculosis usually occurs at an early age. Although often asymptomatic with no clinical signs, it may cause a mild febrile illness, **erythema nodosum** (painful, indurated shin lesions) and small pleural effusions. Bronchial compression by lymphadenopathy may cause wheeze and occasionally lobar collapse followed by late **bronchiectasis** (Chapter 30).

Post-primary tuberculosis develops over months, with malaise, anorexia, weight loss, night sweats and a productive cough. Breathlessness, chest pain, haemoptysis and cervical lymphadenopathy may occur. Clinical signs of pneumonia and pleural effusion are common, whereas lupus vulgaris (an indolent skin infection) is less frequent. **Miliary tuberculosis** presents with a non-specific pyrexial illness, malaise and weight loss. Sparse clinical signs include hepatomegaly and choroidal tubercles in the retina.

Investigation

Blood tests may detect anaemia, decreased sodium and increased calcium.

Mantoux test: strongly positive in post-primary pulmonary tuberculosis (>5 mm skin induration with 10 units of intradermal tuberculin injection). The test is often negative in miliary TB (reduced host response) and HIV-infected patients (reduced cellular immunity).

Heaf test (screening test): A ring of six pinpricks is made through a tuberculin solution placed on the forearm. No response at 4–7 days (grade 0) demonstrates lack of immunity; four to six discrete nodules (grade 1) or a ring formed by coalition of the six pinpricks (grade 2) indicate immunity. A single nodule formed by infilling of the ring (grade 3) represents recent contact or early tuberculous infection, and a nodule >5–7 mm with surface vesicles or ulceration (grade 4) suggests infection.

Microbiology: the acid-fast bacilli may be detected in sputum or lung washings using the Ziehl–Neelsen stain. However, bacilli are slow-growing, and culture and drug sensitivities take 4–6 weeks. Bone marrow or cerebrospinal fluid (CSF) culture may confirm the diagnosis of miliary tuberculosis.

Histopathology: pleural aspiration with biopsy confirms tuberculosis in ~90% of patients with pleural effusions. Liver biopsy will isolate miliary tuberculosis in ~60% of cases.

Chest radiography (Fig. 33b): upper lobe shadowing is suggestive of tuberculosis. Apical cavities, pleural effusions and pneumothoraces may occur. In miliary tuberculosis, widespread small nodules (2–3 mm diameter) are diffusely spread throughout the lungs (miliary shadowing), and are easily missed.

Prevention

Vaccination of non-immune subjects, assessed by Heaf testing at age 12–13, with **BCG** (bacille Calmette–Guérin), a non-virulent strain of bovine TB, produces immunity and reduces the risk of pulmonary tuberculosis by 70%.

Drug therapy

The prognosis in tuberculosis is good if the patient is not immunocompromised. Good nutrition, reduced alcohol consumption and **compliance with drug therapy** are important factors in successful treatment. Uncomplicated pulmonary tuberculosis is treated for 6 months. Initially, at least three drugs are used, to prevent the development of resistant strains. The recommended regime is rifampicin, pyrazinamide and isoniazid for 2 months, followed by rifampicin and isoniazid for 4 months. Additional pyridoxine prevents isoniazid-induced peripheral neuropathy. Liver function tests should be monitored, as rifampicin and pyrazinamide can cause liver dysfunction. If drug resistance is suspected (TB recurrence in a non-compliant patient) then a four-drug regimen (adding ethambutol) may be initiated. When culture results are available, alternative drugs replace those to which the mycobacterium is not sensitive. Ethambutol (monitor colour vision for optic neuritis), streptomycin (monitor plasma levels to avoid hearing impairment) or ciprofloxacin may be used.

In some organs (e.g. bone), tuberculosis is treated for longer, often with additional drugs. In meningeal or cerebral tuberculosis, a four-drug regime for 12 months with additional steroids is recommended, to ensure adequate brain penetration and to prevent cranial nerve compression by meningeal scarring.

Complications

Reactivation of old tuberculous scars may occur when a patient is immunocompromised (Fig. 33c). Chemoprophylaxis with isoniazid is often given before immunosuppressive treatment (chemotherapy, organ transplantation). Bronchiectasis and lung cavities with secondary fungal infections (mycetoma), cranial nerve lesions and renal tract obstructions may develop due to scarring associated with healing after tuberculosis. Surgery may be required to correct these defects. Non-compliance or inadequate treatment results in multiresistant strains of mycobacteria that may be very difficult to eradicate. Compulsory supervision and isolation of these patients may be required.

Contact tracing

Community health services **must be notified** when a patient is diagnosed with TB, to trace contacts and prevent spread of the disease. Contacts are screened with a Heaf test. If this suggests a risk of infection, then chest radiography and appropriate follow-up is arranged.

34 Respiratory infections in HIV infection

(a) Common respiratory infections in HIV-infected individuals

Microbe	Typical CD4$^+$ cell count (per mm^3)
Bacteria	
S. pneumoniae	Any
Haemophilus species	Any
P. aeruginosa	<200
L. pneumophila	Any
Mycobacteria	
M. tuberculosis	Any (extrapulmonary or atypical presentation when <200)
Disseminated MAC	<50
Fungi	
Pneumocystis carinii	<200
Cryptococcus neoformans	<200
Histoplasma capsulatum	<200
Coccidiodes immitis	<100
Virus	
Cytomegalovirus	<50

(b) CXR of pneumocystis carinii pneumonia, showing diffuse alveolar infilftrate

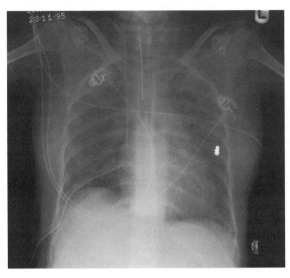

Respiratory complications of human immunodeficiency virus (HIV) infection are related to the **degree of immunosuppression** and the **development of acquired immune deficiency syndrome (AIDS)**. Highly active antiretroviral therapy (**HAART**) allows expansion of the immune system and has improved the survival of patients with AIDS, partly by decreasing the rate of respiratory infection. Nevertheless, HIV-infected individuals are at increased risk of infection with **mycobacteria, *Pneumocystis carinii*,** or **other fungi** (Fig. 34a).

Pneumocystis carinii pneumonia (PCP) remains a common cause of respiratory illness in patients with HIV, despite the widespread use of prophylaxis. PCP rarely occurs in Africa, however; it seems to be a disease of developed countries. PCP may be transmitted via inhalation rather than by reactivation of dormant infection. Patients with PCP have progressive dyspnoea on exertion, malaise, fever, non-productive cough and hypoxia. In contrast to patients with other causes of immunosuppression, PCP in the HIV-infected is indolent over weeks. Radiographs usually show diffuse interstitial infiltrates early and alveolar infiltrates late (Fig. 34b). **Spontaneous pneumothorax** (Chapter 29) is common, particularly in patients receiving aerosolized prophylaxis. PCP rarely occurs in patients with CD4$^+$ cell (Chapter 17) counts >300/mm^3, and most patients have counts <100/mm^3. Diagnosis requires demonstration of **cysts** or **trophozoites** in induced sputum or bronchoalveolar lavage. Trimethoprim-sulfamethoxazole is the most effective therapy. Corticosteroids are co-administered to patients with hypoxaemia to avoid respiratory deterioration often observed in the first days of therapy.

Bacterial pneumonias (Chapter 32) are extremely common in patients with HIV infection just as in immunocompetent patients. *Streptococcus pneumoniae* and *Haemophilus influenzae* are most common, but in many communities, *Staphylococcus aureus* and *Pseudomonas aeruginosa* are also common. Symptoms, signs and radiographs are generally similar to those in immunocompetent patients (Chapter 32). The presence of high fever, purulent sputum, rapid onset of symptoms or pleuritic chest pain help distinguish bacterial pneumonia from PCP. *Legionella* infections are more common in patients with HIV infection.

Mycobacterial infections from *Mycobacterium tuberculosis* (MTB) or *M. avium complex* (MAC) are significant concerns in patients with HIV. Approximately one-third of HIV-infected patients exposed to MTB will develop primary disease, and patients with prior exposure have a 10%/year chance of developing reactivation disease. **Tuberculin skin tests** should be performed on all patients with HIV infection. Induration of >5 mm is consistent with prior MTB infection, and requires prophylactic treatment in the absence of active disease. False-negative tuberculin reactions are usual once CD4+ counts are <100/mm^3. The clinical manifestations of MTB infection depend on the degree of immunosuppression. When CD4+ counts are >300/mm^3, the clinical presentation is similar to that in patients without HIV infection, including fever, non-productive cough and upper lobe cavitary disease. As immunosuppression advances, **mediastinal adenopathy, diffuse or miliary pulmonary infiltrates,** and extrapulmonary (**nodal, bone marrow, genitourinary, central nervous system**) involvement become more typical. Patients with MTB treated with HAART may develop worsening systemic symptoms, fever and adenopathy due to immune reconstitution. HIV-infected patients with MTB should receive the standard drug therapy for their community for ≥9 months. The high prevalence of MTB disease in patients with HIV infection has contributed to the spread of **multidrug resistance** in many regions.

MAC infection presents as a disseminated systemic wasting disease in patients with CD4+ cell counts <50/mm^3. Patients have malaise, fever, night sweats, abdominal pain, diarrhea, weight loss or non-productive cough. **Anaemia** and **elevated alkaline phosphatase** are the most common laboratory abnormalities. Radiographs are often normal, or have nodular infiltrates. The use of prophylactic antibiotics in patients with low CD4+ cell counts is effective in reducing the risk of disseminated MAC infection.

Other fungal infections: the combined humoral and cellular immunodeficiency due to HIV infection also leads to an increased risk of infection due to **fungi**, many which are ubiquitous in the environment. Most fungal infections cause disease predominantly outside the respiratory tract but respiratory symptoms are not unusual. *Cryptococcus* often has concurrent respiratory manifestations with meningitis. Respiratory symptoms are non-specific, and radiographs usually show interstitial or nodular infiltrates. Culturing fungus or demonstration of cryptococcal antigen in blood and CSF are diagnostic. In endemic areas, **histoplasmosis** and **coccidioidomycosis** may cause respiratory disease in HIV-infected individuals. Both cause a systemic illness with fever, weight loss, dyspnoea, and non-productive cough. Coccidioidomycosis is usually seen in patients with CD4+ cell counts <300/mm^3. Radiographic abnormalities range from diffuse alveolar/interstitial infiltrates to localized nodules/masses or adenopathy. Diagnosis requires stain or culture of the fungus. Blood cultures are usually positive in cases of histoplasmosis.

Cytomegalovirus (CMV) is a major cause of pneumonia in patients immunosuppressed after organ transplantation, but it is not a major respiratory pathogen in HIV-infected individuals. CMV is often recovered in respiratory samples by culture or antigen detection, but it does not cause primary pneumonia until CD4+ cell counts are very low. More commonly, CMV is found in conjunction with another pathogen. Diagnosis of CMV pneumonitis in an HIV-infected individual requires evidence of parenchymal invasion or cytopathological effect in a symptomatic patient without evidence of other infection.

Malignancies involving the respiratory system may be confused with infections in HIV-infected individuals. **Kaposi's sarcoma (KS)** and **non-Hodgkin's lymphoma** (NHL) are the most common malignancies. KS is a tumour of vascular origin related to infection with **human herpesvirus 8**. Patients with lung involvement usually have concurrent skin or upper respiratory tract involvement. Its clinical manifestations range from an asymptomatic incidental finding on radiograph to fulminant disease causing respiratory failure. NHL in the lung may present radiographically as nodules, mass(es), or effusions. Symptoms are typical of a systemic or respiratory illness. NHL typically occurs in patients with advanced immunosuppression and CD4+ cell counts <100/mm^3. NHLs are typically aggressive B-cell or Burkitt's lymphoma, suggesting a relationship with pre-existing herpesvirus infections. HIV-infected individuals may be at greater risk of developing **advanced lung cancer** at young age, with a poor prognosis for survival. Many of these patients have early HIV infection without a history of opportunistic infection.

35 Acute respiratory distress syndrome (ARDS)

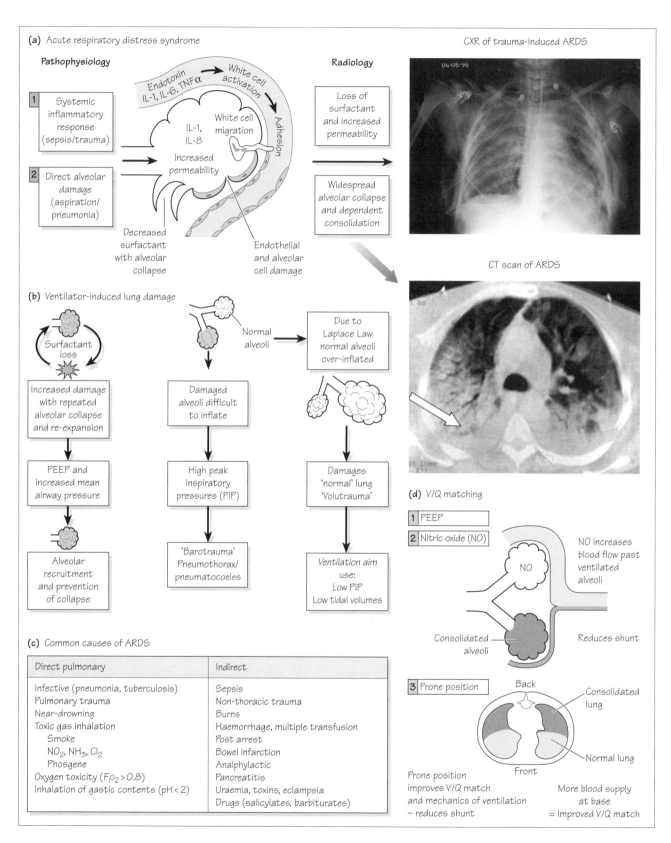

(a) Acute respiratory distress syndrome

Pathophysiology

Endotoxin IL-1, IL-6, TNFα → White cell activation → Adhesion

1 Systemic inflammatory response (sepsis/trauma)

2 Direct alveolar damage (aspiration/ pneumonia)

IL-1, IL-8
Increased permeability
White cell migration

Decreased surfactant with alveolar collapse

Endothelial and alveolar cell damage

Radiology

Loss of surfactant and increased permeability

Widespread alveolar collapse and dependent consolidation

CXR of trauma-induced ARDS

CT scan of ARDS

(b) Ventilator-induced lung damage

Surfactant loss

Increased damage with repeated alveolar collapse and re-expansion

PEEP and increased mean airway pressure

Alveolar recruitment and prevention of collapse

Normal alveoli → Due to Laplace Law normal alveoli over-inflated

Damaged alveoli difficult to inflate

High peak inspiratory pressures (PIP)

'Barotrauma' Pneumothorax/ pneumatocoeles

Damages 'normal' lung 'Volutrauma'

Ventilation aim use: Low PIP Low tidal volumes

(d) V/Q matching

1 PEEP

2 Nitric oxide (NO)

NO

NO increases blood flow past ventilated alveoli

Consolidated alveoli

Reduces shunt

3 Prone position

Back
Consolidated lung
Normal lung
Front

Prone position improves V/Q match and mechanics of ventilation – reduces shunt

More blood supply at base = Improved V/Q match

(c) Common causes of ARDS

Direct pulmonary	Indirect
Infective (pneumonia, tuberculosis)	Sepsis
Pulmonary trauma	Non-thoracic trauma
Near-drowning	Burns
Toxic gas inhalation	Haemorrhage, multiple transfusion
Smoke	Post arrest
NO_2, NH_3, Cl_2	Bowel infarction
Phosgene	Analphylactic
Oxygen toxicity ($F_iO_2 > 0.8$)	Pancreatitis
Inhalation of gastic contents (pH < 2)	Uraemia, toxins, eclampsia
	Drugs (salicylates, barbiturates)

ARDS is most simply defined as 'leaky lung syndrome' or 'low pressure (i.e. non-cardiogenic) pulmonary oedema'. It describes an acute, diffuse inflammatory lung injury, often in previously healthy lungs (Fig. 35a) in response to a variety of direct (i.e. inhaled) or indirect (i.e. blood borne) insults.

The **internationally agreed criteria** for diagnosis of ARDS are:
1 Severe hypoxaemia, $P_aO_2/F_IO_2 < 200$, (+/–PEEP) e.g. P_aO_2 (55 mmHg)/F_IO_2 (80% inspired O_2) = 55/0.8 = (75).
2 Bilateral diffuse pulmonary infiltrates on chest X-ray.
3 Normal or only slightly elevated left atrial pressure (pulmonary artery occlusion pressure <18 mmHg).
Acute lung injury (ALI) is the precursor to ARDS. Apart from a lesser degree of hypoxaemia ($P_aO_2/F_IO_2 < 300$), the criteria for diagnosis are the same.

Epidemiology and prognosis

The **incidence** of ARDS is ~2–8 cases per 100 000 population per year, but its precursor ALI is much commoner. ARDS mortality is generally **high (>50%)** but is determined by the precipitating condition (~35% for trauma, ~60% for sepsis, and ~80% for aspiration pneumonia). Age (>60 years) and sepsis are also associated with increased mortality. Early diagnosis and treatment may improve outcome. The cause of death is **multiorgan failure (MOF)**, usually due to a combination of tissue hypoxia and overwhelming secondary infection. Less than 20% of patients die from hypoxaemia alone.

Pathogenesis (Fig. 35a) and causes (Fig. 35c)

During the **acute inflammatory phase** of ARDS, cytokine-activated neutrophils and monocytes adhere to pulmonary endothelium or alveolar epithelium, releasing inflammatory mediators and proteolytic enzymes (Chapter 17). These damage the integrity of the alveolar–capillary membrane, increase permeability and cause alveolar oedema. Reduced surfactant production causes alveolar collapse and hyaline membrane formation. The loss of functioning alveoli and ventilation/perfusion mismatch leads to progressive hypoxaemia and respiratory failure. The subsequent late **healing fibroproliferative phase** results in progressive pulmonary fibrosis and reduced compliance (stiff lungs). Associated pulmonary hypertension is partially due to activation of the coagulation cascade, with pulmonary capillary microthrombosis and regional hypoxic vasoconstriction.

Clinical features

The **acute inflammatory phase** lasts 3–10 days and results in hypoxaemia and MOF. It presents with progressive breathlessness, tachypnoea, central cyanosis, hypoxic confusion and lung crepitations. These symptoms and signs are in no way diagnostic and are shared with many other pulmonary conditions. During the later **healing, fibroproliferative phase**, pulmonary fibrosis (lung scaring) and pneumothoraces (Chapter 29) are common. Secondary chest and systemic infections complicate both phases.

Investigation

Monitoring: routine measurements include temperature, respiratory rate, O_2 saturation and urine output. In addition, the arterial and central venous pressures, the cardiac output and occasionally the left atrial pressure (using a pulmonary artery catheter) are measured **to assess fluid balance and ensure adequate tissue oxygen delivery**. Serial blood gas measurements are used to monitor gas exchange. Early detection of secondary pulmonary infection requires microbiological examination of sputum or bronchoalveolar washings. **Radiological:** serial CXRs identify progression of **diffuse bilateral pulmonary infiltrates**. Similarly, early computed tomography (CT) scanning can identify **diffuse patchy infiltrates** with **dependent consolidation**; later scans reveal **pneumothoraces, pneumatoceles** and fibrosis.

Management

The key to successful management of ARDS is to **establish and treat the underlying cause**. In the early stages, oxygen therapy and physiotherapy may suffice. With progressive respiratory failure, non-invasive ventilation — with continuous positive airway pressure (CPAP) or non-invasive positive pressure ventilation (NIPPV) — or full mechanical ventilation and high-inspired oxygen concentrations may be required to maintain adequate ventilation and oxygenation. The high airways pressures needed to achieve normal tidal volumes during mechanical ventilation often result in lung damage (barotrauma), including pneumothorax and lung cysts. This ventilator-induced lung injury and oxygen toxicity ($F_IO_2 > 0.8$) must be prevented, as these contribute to mortality and MOF.

The basic principles of mechanical ventilation are to **limit pressure-induced damage, optimize oxygenation** and **avoid circulatory compromise** (reduced cardiac output and blood pressure due to high intrathoracic pressures; see also Chapter 38). A 'protective lung ventilation strategy' of low tidal volumes (6 mL/kg) and low peak inspiratory pressures (<30 cmH$_2$O) reduce lung damage, complications and mortality. **Alveolar recruitment** (of collapsed alveoli) is achieved with high positive end-expiratory pressures (PEEP >10 cm H$_2$O) or long inspiratory-to-expiratory times. The CO_2 retention ('permissive hypercapnia') resulting from this strategy of low tidal volume ventilation can be tolerated for long periods.

Excessive fluid loading must be avoided, as this increases the alveolar flooding characteristic of ARDS. The aim must be to maintain adequate perfusion of other organs whilst using the lowest possible left atrial pressures. In the acute situation, diuretics may be essential to correct hypoxaemia by reducing extravascular lung water. Thereafter, combinations of pulmonary and systemic vasodilators (before and after load reduction of the left heart), inotropes and vasoconstrictor agents may be used to achieve adequate cardiac output and perfusion pressures at low left atrial filling pressures.

Essential general measures include good nursing care, physiotherapy, nutrition and infection control. Reducing fever (shivering) and controlling anxiety with sedation decreases metabolic demand. **No drug therapy has been consistently beneficial** in early ARDS, including steroids, anti-inflammatory agents, anticytokines or surfactant therapy. However, 7–10 days after onset, steroid therapy may prevent the development of subsequent pulmonary fibrosis. **Inhaled nitric oxide** and nursing the patient in the **prone position** improves gas exchange by increasing perfusion to ventilated areas of lung, but no survival benefit has been demonstrated (Fig. 35d). **Extracorporeal membrane oxygenation (ECMO)** techniques to oxygenate blood or remove CO_2 are effective in children, but the benefit in adults has not been established.

36 Lung cancer

(a) Mass on CT: A>3 cm spiculated mass is seen in upper lobe of the right lung

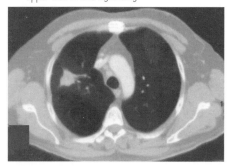

(b) Fibreoptic bronchoscopy showing tumour invading bronchus

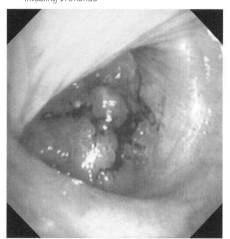

(c) CXR showing squamous cell tumour in hilar region

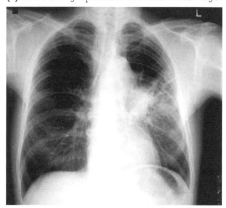

(d) Staging system for non-small cell lung cancers

Stage	T (tumour)	N (node)	M (metastasis)	Key
IA	T1	N0	M0	**T1:** ≤3 cm without division
IB	T2	N0	M0	**T2:** >3 cm, or invasion of main bronchus
IIA	T1	N1	M0	>2 cm from main carina, or invades
IIB	T2	N1	M0	visceral pleura, or bronchus causing
	T3	N0	M0	obstruction
				T3: Invades chest wall or pleura, or main bronchus <2 cm from main carina
				T4: Invades adjacent structure, malignant effusion, satellite nodules
IIIA	T1, 2, 3	N2	M0	**N0:** No lymph node metastasis
	T3	N1	M0	**N1:** Ipsilateral hilar lymph nodes
IIIB	T1, 2, 3, 4	N3	M0	**N2:** Ipsilateral mediastinal or subcarinal lymph nodes
	T4	N1, 2	M0	**N3:** Contralateral, scalene or supra-clavicular lymph nodes
IV	T1–4	N0–3	M1	**M0:** No distant metastasis
				M1: Any distant metastasis

(e) Survival for non-small cell cancer

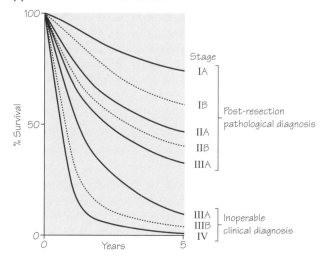

More people die in the US and Europe from **lung cancer** than from breast, prostate and colon cancer combined. Furthermore, the number of cases is likely to increase in the next 25 years due to continued use of cigarettes, particularly in women. Lung cancer has a **worse prognosis** than other common cancers, with an overall **5-year survival** of **13%**.

Risks

Cigarette smoking accounts for the vast majority of lung cancer cases. Risk is directly related to the duration and number of cigarettes smoked, age of initiation, depth of inhalation and levels of tar and nicotine. In heavy smokers (>20 pack-years) the lifetime risk of lung cancer is 10%, 10–30 times greater than for lifelong non-smokers (<0.3%). After quitting cigarettes, risk gradually declines over 15 years, but remains 2–5 times greater than in non-smokers. **Passive smoking** in non-smokers may increase the risk by ~1.5%.

Asbestos exposure is the most common occupational risk for lung cancer (Chapter 31). Tobacco smoke is synergistic with asbestosis, increasing the relative risk to 6–60 times that of a non-smoker. **Radon gas**, found naturally in rocks, soil and ground water, may also increase risk.

Classification

Lung cancers are divided pathologically into **small cell** (**SC**, 20–30% of total) and **non-small cell** (**NSC**, 70–80% of total) types. NSC types are grouped due to their similar biology, treatment and prognosis, and include **squamous cell** (30%), **large cell** (15%), and **adenocarcinoma** (33%), which is increasing in prevalence, especially in women. **Adenocarcinomas** typically present as a peripheral nodule (<3 cm) or mass (>3 cm); they are the most common type in non-smokers, and mainly arise in areas of pulmonary scarring. Bronchoalveolar cell carcinoma is an adenocarcinoma variant with low metastatic potential. **Squamous cell carcinomas** arise from the bronchial epithelium, and generally present as a central mass with tumour visible in the airway (Fig. 36a,b), often with symptoms due to local tumour invasion (cough, haemoptysis, chest pain and hoarseness). **Large cell carcinoma** is undifferentiated, and lacks the histological features of adenocarcinoma or squamous cell carcinoma; it generally presents as a large peripheral mass, often with metastases. **SC** carcinomas arise from neuroendocrine cells in the bronchial submucosa, and typically present as a central mass with lymph-node enlargement. These are aggressive tumours that invade lymphatics and blood vessels. Nearly all have metastasized at diagnosis.

Presentation

Less than 10% of lung cancers are discovered incidentally in asymptomatic patients. Most patients are 50–70 years of age, with non-specific symptoms including new unresolving cough, haemoptysis, chest pain, hoarseness, dyspnoea on exertion, malaise and weight loss. Symptoms due to haematogenous **extrathoracic metastasis** to bone, liver, bone marrow, adrenals and brain are present in around one-third of patients at diagnosis.

Paraneoplastic syndromes—signs or symptoms associated with lung cancers that are not related directly to metastatic tumour—may precede radiographic demonstration. They may be due to secretion of hormones or hormone-like substances from tumours, or serum **autoantibodies** (e.g. anti-Hu) related to tumour antigens. SC carcinoma is associated with most paraneoplastic syndromes including Cushing's syndrome, syndrome of inappropriate secretion of anti-diuretic hormone (SIADH), Lambert–Eaton syndrome, cerebellar ataxia, or idiopathic orthostatic hypotension. Squamous cell cancer may cause hypercalcaemia from release of parathyroid hormone-related peptide.

Physical findings in the lung are related to disease extent. Small **parenchymal nodules** are undetectable by physical examination. Focal findings may be due to atelectasis, airway invasion, pleural effusion (Chapter 28) or supraclavicular adenopathy. Invasion of adjacent structures may cause superior vena cava syndrome (obstruction), Horner's syndrome (autonomic overactivity), or brachial plexopathy. Digital clubbing or hypertrophic pulmonary osteoarthropathy may be present.

Evaluation

Evaluation of patients with suspected lung cancer should include demonstration of **malignancy**, **staging** and **suitability for therapy**. Radiographs provide information regarding the size and location of the tumour, benign calcification, involvement of adjacent structures, atelectasis, pleural effusion, and adenopathy (Fig. 36c). **Computed tomography** (**CT**) **scans** are superior to plain X-rays. If a focal lesion does not change in two years, it is unlikely to be malignant. **Positron emission tomography** (**PET**) **scanning** has a high sensitivity for distinguishing benign from malignant nodules and for detecting nodal or distant metastases.

Staging is assessment of the extent of the tumour, and largely determines treatment options and prognosis. Separate staging systems are used for SC and NSC cancers. **SC cancer** is staged as either **limited** or **extensive** disease. **Limited disease** describes tumour confined to one hemithorax, including malignant pleural effusion and supraclavicular lymph node metastasis. **Extensive disease** describes metastatic spread beyond the hemithorax. SC cancer is generally an incurable disease. Standard therapy for limited disease (33%) is combination chemotherapy and radiotherapy, with response rates approaching 90%; median survival with therapy is ~18 months. Standard therapy for extensive disease (66%) is chemotherapy. The response rate is ~70%, treatment prolonging median survival from ~3 months to ~1 year.

NSC cancer staging is based on the **tumour** (T), **node** (N), and **metastasis** (M) classification system (Fig. 36d). **T3** tumours invade thoracic structures that are potentially resectable, and **T4** tumours include malignant effusions or tumours invading non-resectable structures. Summation of **TNM categories** determines the stage of disease and treatment, and predicts survival (Fig. 36e). In functional patients with **stage I** or **II** disease and adequate pulmonary reserve (postoperative FEV_1 >800 mL), **surgical resection** is optimal. Some patients with **stage IIIA** disease are surgical candidates. Patients with **stage IIIB** or **IV** disease are not candidates for curative resection. Unresectable disease is generally treated with **chemotherapy** and **radiation therapy**, or radiation alone. **Stage IV** disease is incurable (median survival 6–12 months). Treatment options are palliative. Painful bone metastases, brain metastasis, or airway obstruction may improve with directed therapy. The benefit of aggressive chemotherapy for patients with advanced disease is modest. **Platinum** and **taxol-based** chemotherapy regimens are currently most common for NSC cancer.

37 Sleep-disordered breathing

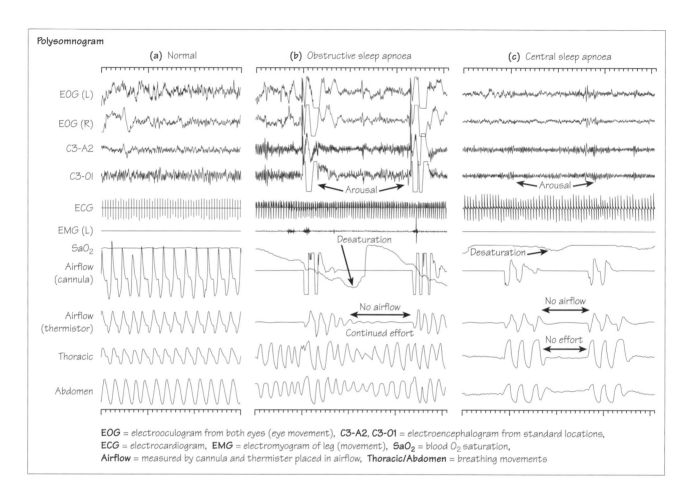

Polysomnogram

(a) Normal **(b)** Obstructive sleep apnoea **(c)** Central sleep apnoea

EOG (L)
EOG (R)
C3-A2
C3-O1
ECG
EMG (L)
SaO₂
Airflow (cannula)
Airflow (thermistor)
Thoracic
Abdomen

Arousal — Arousal

Desaturation — Desaturation

No airflow — No airflow

Continued effort — No effort

EOG = electrooculogram from both eyes (eye movement), **C3-A2, C3-O1** = electroencephalogram from standard locations,
ECG = electrocardiogram, **EMG** = electromyogram of leg (movement), **SaO₂** = blood O_2 saturation,
Airflow = measured by cannula and thermister placed in airflow, **Thoracic/Abdomen** = breathing movements

Sleep-disordered breathing is a common problem, with a vast potential for improvement in the patient's quality of life. Normal sleep (Fig. 37) consists of rapid eye movement (**REM**) and non-rapid eye movement (**NREM**) sleep. REM sleep normally comprises about 25–30% of total sleep, and is characterized by an awake-pattern electroencephalography (EEG), voluntary muscle atonia and dreaming. NREM sleep is divided into **light (Stages 1, 2)** and **deep (Stages 3,4)** sleep. Ventilatory drive is normally diminished in REM compared to NREM sleep, causing a slight fall in P_aO_2 and a rise in P_aCO_2, the magnitude of changes depending on starting conditions. Normal duration and architecture of sleep results in the absence of daytime **hypersomnolence**, which can be quantified by sleep latency or wakefulness testing. Daytime hypersomnolence due to sleep deprivation and sleep fragmentation may lead to an overall decrease in quality of life, including increased risk of motor vehicle accidents and cognitive dysfunction. It may be due to a variety of causes, including **obstructive sleep apnoea** and more rarely **central sleep apnoea**.

Sleep-disordered breathing is diagnosed using **polysomnography** (Fig. 37), which records the EEG for sleep patterns, movements of abdomen and thorax to assess breathing, oronasal flow and oximetry for O_2 saturation.

Obstructive sleep apnoea (OSA) is characterized by the absence of airflow with continued respiratory effort (Fig. 37b). Up to 4% of the general population and approximately 90% of patients with sleep apnoea have OSA. OSA is far more common in males than females, and is associated with alcohol consumption, increasing age, obesity, increased neck circumference, hypertension and hypothyroidism. Obstruction typically occurs in the upper airway and pharynx, and is related to the normal decreases in upper airway muscle tone and increased airway resistance that occur in deep or REM sleep. It may also occur in children with inflamed or enlarged tonsils or adenoids. These factors, in conjunction with individual anatomy, extraluminal tissue and posture, result in airway collapse/closure during inspiration, when airway pressure is reduced. Apnoea resolves with arousal and restoration of muscle tone. Although many hundreds or thousands of episodes of apnoea and arousal may occur each night, patients are often unaware of them; their sleep partners commonly report **loud snoring**, snorting or apnoea. Patients develop **daytime hypersomnolence**, **loud snoring** and **weight gain**. Their physical examination may demonstrate pedal oedema, nasal congestion, enlarged tongue, shallow palate, enlarged uvula or retrognathia. Most patients have normal arterial blood gases and haemoglobin. In chronic obstructive pulmonary disease (COPD) patients, **nocturnal hypoxia** can be severe even with mild OSA, and gas exchange is already compromised and they may be already hypoxaemic with a low O_2 saturation.

In OSA, polysomnography reveals repeated episodes of OSA or hypopnoea (reduced flow with oxygen desaturation or arousal), which terminate with arousal (Fig. 37b). These episodes are quantified by the **apnoea plus hypopnoea index** (**AHI**, episodes/h). Normal sleep may have an AHI < 10. Severe OSA usually has an AHI > 40. A minority of patients with very severe OSA may de-velop **obesity hypoventilation syndrome** (Pickwick syndrome). Obstructive episodes can cause **pulmonary hypertension** (Chapter 24) from hypoxic pulmonary vasoconstriction. Systemic blood pressure increases during apnoeas, possibly due to sympathetic stimulation, and LV afterload increases during obstructive apnoeas due to the marked fall in pleural pressure during episodes. There is a strong association between OSA and daytime systemic hypertension, although causality has not been established.

Therapy for OSA requires relief of obstruction. Moderate weight loss (≥10%) will often result in substantial improvement in patients with mild OSA. **Nasal continuous positive airway pressure** (**CPAP**, Chapter 38) is the most commonly prescribed therapy, and is effective in compliant patients. Unfortunately, about 50% of patients will not comply with nasal CPAP long-term. Some patients will respond to oral appliances or uvulopalatopharyngoplasty (surgery). Tracheostomy bypasses the obstruction, and will relieve OSA; however, it is associated with psychological and local compli-

cations. O_2 alone may decrease or eliminate hypoxia, but will not treat obstruction or eliminate arousals.

Central sleep apnoea (**CSA**) is characterized by cessation of air-flow during sleep without evidence of respiratory effort, and is due to a **loss or inhibition of central respiratory drive** (Fig. 37c). Patients with CSA may be subdivided into those with daytime hypercapnia or normocapnia. CSA with daytime hypercapnia is usually due to central alveolar hypoventilation, neuromuscular disease or chest wall disease (e.g. kyphoscoliosis). Central alveolar hypoventilation may be primary (Ondine's curse) or secondary to brainstem disease (see Chapter 11). Neuromuscular causes include muscular dystrophy, phrenic nerve dysfunction, myositis (muscle inflammation) and myasthenia gravis. Patients with a CNS cause for hypoventilation ('won't breathe') may benefit from a respiratory stimulant. Patients with weakness or chest wall disease ('can't breathe') benefit from assisted mechanical ventilation. **Positive pressure ventilation** with a nasal or face mask is most commonly prescribed (Chapter 38). Tracheostomy with assisted positive pressure ventilation is also effective.

Cheyne–Stokes breathing (**CSB**) is characterized by oscillatory ventilation due to instability in ventilatory control. During sleep, patients will alternate periods of hyperpnoea with hypopnoea/apnoea. CSB is most commonly due to congestive heart failure or neurological disease. CSB may be treated with O_2, respiratory stimulants (theophylline) or assisted ventilation. Congestive heart failure related CSB improves with diuretics and afterload reduction.

38 Mechanical ventilation

(a) Indications for mechanical ventilation or support in adults

Surgery General anaesthesia with neuromuscular blockade Post-operative management following major surgery	Cervical cord damage above C4 Neck fractures
Respiratory centre depression Usually when Pa_{CO_2} >7–8 kPa (50–60 mmHg) Head injury Drug overdose: e.g. opiates, barbiturates Raised intracranial pressure: cerebral haemorrhage/ tumours/meningitis/encephalitis Status epilepticus	Neuromuscular disorders – when VC <20–30 mL/kg Guillain–Barré Myasthenia gravis Poliomyelitis Polyneuritis
	Chest wall disorders Kyphoscoliosis Trauma: especially flail segment (multiple rib fractures → section of chest wall unattached)
Lung disease Pneumonia Acute respiratory distress syndrome (ARDS) Severe asthma attack Acute exacerbation of chronic obstructive pulmonary disease (COPD), cystic fibrosis Trauma–lung contusion Pulmonary oedema	Other Cardiac arrest Severe circulatory shock Resistant hypoxia in Type 1 respiratory failure (reduces oxygen consumption)

(b) Nasal mask and NIPPV

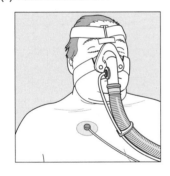

(c) Airway pressure profiles in different types of ventilation

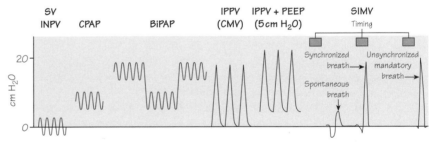

SV = spontaneous ventilation, **INPV** = intermittent negative pressure ventilation, **CPAP** = continuous positive airway pressure, **BiPAP** = biphasic continuous positive airway pressure, **IPPV** = intermittent positive pressure ventilation (= **CMV**), **CMV** = controlled mechanical ventilation, **PEEP** = positive end-expiratory pressure, **SIMV** = synchronized intermittent mandatory ventilation. If a spontaneous breath occurs in the timing window it triggers a synchronized ventilator breath and if not a mandatory breath is given soon after the timing window.

(d) Complications of mechanical ventilation

Risks during endotracheal intubation or tracheostomy Myocardial depression from anaesthetic Aspiration of gastric contents Fall in Pa_{O_2} during apnoea Reflex bronchoconstriction and laryngospasm	Risks associated with sedation and paralysis Cardiac depression Depression of respiratory drive (delays weaning) Increases danger of disconnection/ventilator failure
Risks of endotracheal intubation and tracheostomy Intubation of the oesophagus Intubation of a bronchus Blockage/accidental extubation Laryngeal/tracheal damage or stenosis Infection	Risks associated with mechanical ventilation High airway pressure → barotrauma Alveolar overdistension → volutrauma: • Pneumothorax, pneumomediastinum • Subcutaneous emphysema (= air in skin) • Structural damage to lung, airways and capillaries • Bronchopulmonary dysplasia (see Chapter 16)
Risks associated with high inspired oxygen (see Chapter 39)	

Mechanical ventilation is usually used to prevent or treat type 2 respiratory (ventilatory) failure. The main indications in adults are listed in Fig. 38a.

Types of mechanical ventilation (Fig. 38c)

Inspiratory muscle paralysis by poliomyelitis was a common reason for mechanical ventilation in the first half of the 20th century. It was usually performed by **intermittent negative pressure ventilation (INPV)**, which is still occasionally used today. Patients are placed inside a **tank ventilator** sealed at the neck, and tank pressure is intermittently lowered, expanding the chest and lowering intrapleural pressure as in spontaneous breathing. Disadvantages of this 'iron lung' include claustrophobia, discomfort, difficult nursing care and the bulk and expense of the equipment. **Jacket and cuirass ventilators** produce a negative pressure just around the chest, but difficulty in achieving a satisfactory seal limits their use to patients only needing ventilatory augmentation.

From the 1950s, **intermittent positive pressure ventilation (IPPV; controlled mechanical ventilation, CMV)** quickly replaced INPV for most purposes. Air is driven into the lungs by raising airway pressure, usually via an endotracheal or tracheostomy tube. Expiration is achieved by allowing pressure to fall to zero. This simple form of IPPV is used during routine surgery. Typical initial adult settings for IPPV are:

Tidal volume, $V_T = 8–12$ mL/kg

Respiratory frequency, $f = 8–14$ breaths/min

Minute ventilation, $V(= V_T \times f) \approx 6000$ mL/min

Inspiratory time:expiratory time = 1:2–1:3

Minute ventilation is adjusted to maintain $P_a\text{CO}_2$ at about 5 kPa (37 mmHg). A slightly lower $P_a\text{CO}_2$ may be used initially in the presence of raised intracranial pressure. Accepting a higher $P_a\text{CO}_2$ (**permissive hypercapnia**) may prevent the need for excessively high airway pressures. $P_a\text{O}_2$ is maintained above 10 kPa (75 mmHg) by adjusting inspired $F\text{O}_2$. The lowest concentration needed is used, usually in the range 30–60%. It may be preferable to accept a slight lower $P\text{O}_2$ than to use >60% for long periods.

Microprocessor control of ventilators has permitted development of numerous variations of IPPV. For example, in non-paralysed patients, the positive pressure may be synchronized with spontaneous breaths and a mandatory breath given if no spontaneous breaths occur in a preset time (**synchronized intermittent mandatory ventilation, SIMV**). In another form, the ventilator operates only where spontaneous ventilation falls below a preset minimum (**mandatory minute ventilation, MMV**).

If, instead of allowing airway pressure to fall to zero, a small positive pressure is maintained throughout expiration (**positive end-expiratory pressure, PEEP**), there is a reduction in V_A/Q mismatching and an improvement in $P_a\text{O}_2$ in some conditions, such as acute respiratory distress syndrome (ARDS). This occurs because PEEP increases functional residual capacity (FRC) and reduces the closure of airways and alveoli towards the end of expiration. Unfortunately, intrathoracic pressure is raised, impairing venous return, and occasionally the fall in cardiac output can reduce tissue oxygen delivery despite the increased $P_a\text{O}_2$. The increased mean airway pressure caused by PEEP also increases the risk of barotrauma. A good compromise is to use the minimum PEEP required to keep $P\text{O}_2$ at an acceptable level (>8 kPa, 60 mmHg) when breathing 50–60% oxygen.

Non-invasive respiratory support

Non-invasive ventilation avoids the use of tracheal intubation or tracheostomy. An example is INPV (above), but this is no longer widely used. In contrast, non-invasive positive pressure techniques using either a nasal mask (Fig. 38b) or sometimes a full face mask are increasingly being used.

In **continuous positive airway pressure (CPAP)**, a standing pressure of 5–10 cmH_2O is applied to a nasal or face mask in a spontaneously breathing patient (Fig. 38c). This has several potential beneficial effects. First, it helps prevent upper airway collapse in **obstructive sleep apnoea**. In interstitial diseases such as **ARDS**, it recruits alveoli, reducing V_A/Q mismatching. FRC is increased, and this may increase lung compliance by moving the patient onto the steep part of the pressure–volume curve (Chapter 6). CO_2 retention may be a problem during CPAP, and this may be improved by alternating the pressure level between high and low values (**biphasic positive pressure ventilation, BiPAP**) to periodically increase the emptying of the lungs.

CPAP may improve oxygenation and may aid the patient's own respiratory efforts, but it cannot produce ventilation by itself. In contrast, **non-invasive intermittent positive pressure ventilation (NIPPV)** is IPPV delivered by face or, more usually, nasal mask. For it to be used successfully, the patient must be cooperative and introduced to the technique gradually, to allow synchronization of his or her breathing with the ventilator. Its use includes nocturnal ventilation of patients with chronic respiratory failure due to neuromuscular disease or thoracic deformity. It is being used increasingly to treat acute exacerbations of chronic obstructive pulmonary disease (COPD), avoiding the need for intubation and improving survival.

In summary, the main beneficial effect of **CPAP** is recruitment of alveoli. The reduction in collapse sometimes also gives rise to a reduction in the work of breathing. In contrast, **NIPPV** is used to reduce the work of breathing rather than to recruit alveoli. This may be of benefit in the tired (e.g. COPD) patient.

Weaning the patient off the ventilator following surgery is usually achieved by reversing neuromuscular blockade and lightening the anaesthetic level. In intensive-care patients, weaning may be more difficult. Several techniques are used, including removing mechanical ventilation for progressively longer periods, or by using a spontaneously breathing mode (e.g. SIMV), and pressure support in which support is progressively reduced. CPAP applied via the endotracheal tube may also help the weaning process.

Problems are hard to predict accurately, but are most likely following prolonged ventilation, in debilitated patients, or in those with neuromuscular or chronic respiratory disease. A pattern of rapid shallow breathing 5 min after disconnection from the ventilator is one of the more useful predictors of failure.

Complications of mechanical ventilation are numerous, and are listed in Fig. 38d.

39 Acute oxygen therapy

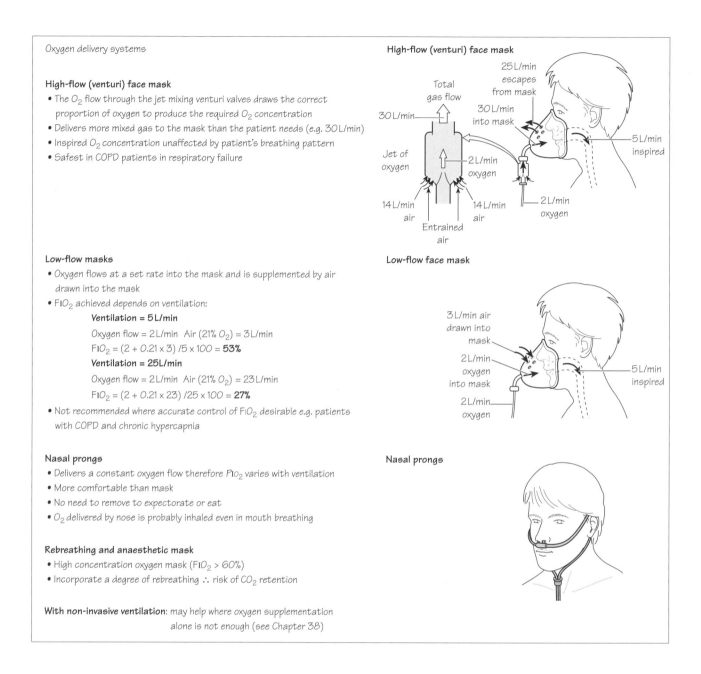

Oxygen delivery systems

High-flow (venturi) face mask
- The O_2 flow through the jet mixing venturi valves draws the correct proportion of oxygen to produce the required O_2 concentration
- Delivers more mixed gas to the mask than the patient needs (e.g. 30 L/min)
- Inspired O_2 concentration unaffected by patient's breathing pattern
- Safest in COPD patients in respiratory failure

Low-flow masks
- Oxygen flows at a set rate into the mask and is supplemented by air drawn into the mask
- FIO_2 achieved depends on ventilation:

    Ventilation = 5 L/min

    Oxygen flow = 2 L/min Air (21% O_2) = 3 L/min

    $FIO_2 = (2 + 0.21 \times 3) / 5 \times 100 = $ **53%**

    Ventilation = 25 L/min

    Oxygen flow = 2 L/min Air (21% O_2) = 23 L/min

    $FIO_2 = (2 + 0.21 \times 23) / 25 \times 100 = $ **27%**

- Not recommended where accurate control of FIO_2 desirable e.g. patients with COPD and chronic hypercapnia

Nasal prongs
- Delivers a constant oxygen flow therefore PIO_2 varies with ventilation
- More comfortable than mask
- No need to remove to expectorate or eat
- O_2 delivered by nose is probably inhaled even in mouth breathing

Rebreathing and anaesthetic mask
- High concentration oxygen mask ($FIO_2 > 60\%$)
- Incorporate a degree of rebreathing ∴ risk of CO_2 retention

With non-invasive ventilation: may help where oxygen supplementation alone is not enough (see Chapter 38)

High-flow (venturi) face mask

Total gas flow

30 L/min

Jet of oxygen

14 L/min air

14 L/min air

Entrained air

25 L/min escapes from mask

30 L/min into mask

2 L/min oxygen

5 L/min inspired

2 L/min oxygen

Low-flow face mask

3 L/min air drawn into mask

2 L/min oxygen into mask

2 L/min oxygen

5 L/min inspired

Nasal prongs

Correctly administered oxygen therapy can be life-saving. The wrong concentration and inadequate monitoring can have severe consequences.

Pathophysiology
Tissues require oxygen for survival. Oxygen utilization is dependent on delivery by the circulation of blood containing adequate quantities of oxygen in a readily releasable form to tissues capable of using the delivered oxygen. **Tissue hypoxia** can be caused by: **low arterial Po_2** (hypoxaemia); inadequate **tissue blood flow** (cardiac failure, emboli); low **haemoglobin concentration** (anaemia); abnormal **oxygen dissociation curve** (haemoglobinopathies, CO poisoning); and **poisoning of intracellular oxygen usage** (e.g. cyanide, sepsis). Tissue hypoxia occurs **within 4 min** of failure of any of these systems, because tissue and lung oxygen reserves are small. Successful treatment requires early recognition, but the clinical features are often non-specific, including altered mental state, dyspnoea, hyperventilation, arrhythmias and hypotension (for details, see Chapter 20). The effects of anaemia and abnormal dissociation curves are discussed in Chapter 8.

Measuring tissue hypoxia

Arterial oxygen saturation (S_aO_2) is measured with a **pulse oximeter**, and partial pressure of oxygen (P_aO_2) by **blood gas analysis**. These are the principal clinical measurements used for initiating, monitoring and adjusting oxygen therapy. However, these measures can be normal when tissue hypoxia is caused by low cardiac output states, anaemia and failure of tissue oxygen use. In these circumstances, **mixed venous oxygen partial pressure** (P_vO_2), which is measured in blood taken from a pulmonary artery catheter, approximates to mean tissue Po_2. Severe hypoxia in a single organ (e.g. due to an arterial embolus) may be associated with a normal P_aO_2, S_aO_2 and P_vO_2. Measurement of individual organ hypoxia is difficult, and requires specialized techniques (e.g. tonometry).

Acute oxygen therapy

The main indications for instituting oxygen therapy are:
Hypoxaemia ($P_aO_2 < 7.8\,kPa$, $S_aO_2 < 90\%$).
Hypotension (systolic blood pressure <100 mmHg).
Low cardiac output and metabolic acidosis (bicarbonate <18 mmol/L).
Respiratory distress (respiratory rate >24/min).
The airway should be checked before starting oxygen therapy, and arterial blood gases analysed as soon as possible to assess P_aO_2, P_aCO_2, pH and bicarbonate.

In the acute situation, the **dose of oxygen may be critical**. Inadequate oxygen accounts for more death and disability than can be justified by the small risks associated with high-dose oxygen. Short periods of high-dose oxygen may preserve life until more specific therapy (e.g. antibiotics, thrombolytics) can be instituted. When blood gas results are available, the dose of oxygen can be adjusted to maintain the P_aO_2 between 8 and 10 kPa. The recommended initial oxygen concentrations as a fraction of oxygen in inspired air (F_iO_2 in percentage) are:
Cardiac or respiratory arrest, 100%.
Hypoxaemia with $P_aCO_2 < 5.3\,kPa$, 40–60%.
Hypoxaemia with $P_aCO_2 > 5.3\,kPa$, initially 24%.
The important features, advantages and disadvantages of different **oxygen delivery systems** are shown in Fig. 39.

Dangers of oxygen therapy

Carbon dioxide retention: high-dose oxygen given to the 10–15% of chronic obstructive pulmonary disease (COPD) patients with type 2 respiratory failure (Chapter 20) will reduce hypoxic drive to breath, increase V/Q mismatching, and may cause CO_2 retention and respiratory acidosis that may be lethal. Fortunately, as these patients are on the steep part of the oxygen dissociation curve, small increases in P_aO_2 cause worthwhile improvements in arterial oxygen content. The initial oxygen concentration should be low (24–28%) and progressively increased if repeat blood gas analysis shows little or no increase in P_aCO_2. The aim is to correct hypoxaemia ($P_aO_2 > 6.65\,kPa$) without decreasing arterial pH below 7.26. Non-invasive positive pressure ventilation and respiratory stimulants may improve ventilation and prevent CO_2 retention. **Pulmonary oxygen toxicity**: $F_iO_2 > 60\%$ may damage the alveolar membrane if inhaled for >24–48 h. **Fire**: facial burns and deaths occur when patients smoke whilst using oxygen. **Absorption collapse**: if an airway becomes blocked, oxygen in the trapped alveolar gas is rapidly absorbed, but N_2 absorption is slow, as alveolar Pn_2 is in equilibrium with mixed venous Pn_2. If N_2 is replaced by O_2 during oxygen therapy, temporary blockage of airways by secretions is more likely to lead to collapsed alveoli, which may be difficult to reopen.

Efficacy of acute oxygen therapy
Arterial hypoxaemia

Right-to-left shunting (e.g. pneumonic consolidation): when shunt is >20%, hypoxia persists despite high F_iO_2.

Alveolar hypoventilation (e.g. drug overdose, neuromuscular disorders): oxygen rapidly corrects hypoxaemia, but the high P_aCO_2 remains. The primary aim is to improve ventilation.

V/Q mismatch (in COPD or asthma, Chapter 14): improved oxygenation, but the response will vary between patients.

Tissue hypoxia without arterial hypoxaemia

Low-output cardiac states (congestive cardiac failure, CCF; myocardial infarction, MI): oxygen solubility is low, and even at F_iO_2 100%, only 30% of total oxygen requirement is carried dissolved in blood. In the absence of hypoxaemia, high oxygen can only marginally improve tissue oxygenation by a small increase in dissolved oxygen. This may preserve some cells with critical oxygen supply, but it must not delay correction of the primary clinical problem (e.g. restoring tissue blood flow).

Chronic lung disease: relief of breathlessness is reported in some patients without hypoxaemia, and a trial of oxygen may be warranted.

Carbon monoxide poisoning: a high F_iO_2 is essential despite a normal P_aO_2, because oxygen competes for haemoglobin binding sites and reduces the half-life of carboxyhaemoglobin from about 320 to 80 min.

Monitoring oxygen therapy

Careful monitoring of oxygen therapy by oximetry (S_aO_2) and arterial blood gas measurement is essential. Oximetry has the advantage of continuous oxygen measurement, whereas blood gases are required to monitor P_aCO_2 and pH.

Stopping oxygen therapy

Oxygen therapy should be stopped when the arterial oxygenation is adequate with the patient breathing room air ($P_aO_2 > 8\,kPa$, $S_aO_2 > 90\%$). In patients without arterial hypoxaemia, oxygen should be stopped when the acid–base state and clinical assessment are consistent with resolution of tissue hypoxia.

Case 1: Asthma

Tom, who is 15 years old, attends his GP's asthma clinic. He has had asthma since early childhood. On two occasions, when he was 8 and 10 years old, he had attacks severe enough to require hospital admission. At present, his asthma is well controlled on regular inhaled beclomethasone dipropionate 200 µg twice daily and inhaled salmeterol 50 µg twice daily. Today, his peak flow is 510 L/min (predicted value for his age and height 530 L/min). On auscultation, there is vesicular breathing and no other sounds.

Questions

1 Is this peak flow normal? Apart from the nomogram values, can you think of any other peak flow reading with which it would be useful to compare today's clinic reading?
2 If you measured the following:
- FEV_1/FVC
- Airway resistance
- Functional residual capacity
- Lung compliance
- Arterial P_{O_2} and arterial P_{CO_2}

—how would they compare with the normal for a boy of his age and size?

On a school trip to a countryside park, Tom becomes a breathless running across a field. His teacher is alarmed by his noisy breathing and asks you, a passing medical student, to assess whether they need to get him to hospital.

3 What simple observations can you make that will help you decide how severe this attack is? In his backpack he has a salbutamol inhaler, a salmeterol inhaler, a sodium cromoglycate inhaler and a beclomethasone inhaler. Which should he use?
4 If you had been able to measure the following during his episode of breathlessness:
- FEV_1/FVC
- Peak flow rate
- Airway resistance
- Functional residual capacity
- Lung compliance
- Arterial P_{O_2} and arterial P_{CO_2}

—how do you think they would they compare with the normal for a boy of his age and size?
5 If you had had your stethoscope with you, what would you have heard on examining his chest?

At 18 years of age, Tom goes to college in London. He stops taking regular medication, as he feels he has 'grown out' of his asthma. He keeps a salbutamol inhaler in his room 'just in case'. During the first term he is well, apart from a couple of wheezy episodes while playing football. In the second term, he develops a heavy cold, and over 24 h he becomes progressively more breathless despite frequent puffs of salbutamol. His friends call out his GP, who finds the following: Tom is fully alert, but talking in broken sentences because he is very breathless. He is not cyanosed. He is using his accessory muscles of respiration. On auscultation, there are wide-spread expiratory rhonchi (wheezes). BP is 115/80, heart rate 110 beats/min, respiratory rate 30 breaths/min, peak flow 200 L/min.

6 Which observations suggest that this is a fairly severe attack?
7 If the GP had measured airway resistance, FRC, lung compliance, arterial P_{O_2} and P_{CO_2}, how would they compare to the predicted values?

His GP decides that this attack warrants hospital admission, and he calls an ambulance. Unfortunately, owing to heavy traffic it is 40 min before he arrives at the local Accident and Emergency Department. By this time, Tom is confused, too breathless to talk and unable to produce a peak flow reading. The casualty officer notices he is now cyanosed, although the widespread rhonchi noted in the GP's letter have now disappeared. Arterial blood gases show arterial $P_{O_2} = 7$ kPa and arterial $P_{CO_2} = 5.5$ kPa while breathing 60% oxygen.

8 Discuss the features which suggest this asthma attack is life-threatening. Do the reduced rhonchi on auscultation contradict the other findings?
9 What is the cause of the low arterial P_{O_2}? Was the inhaled oxygen helpful, and if so was the correct concentration used? Is this P_{CO_2} normal, and how does it affect your assessment of the severity of this attack?

Case 2: Severe breathlessness

A 38-year-old man is seen for evaluation of severe exertional dyspnoea. Two years ago, he had been able to play squash regularly, but he stopped 6 months ago because of dyspnoea and fatigue during exercise. He now reports dyspnoea after climbing one flight of stairs. He has no cough, sputum or wheeze. He smoked one pack of cigarettes a day for 10 years and quit 7 years ago. He has no allergies or pets, and has not travelled outside of Europe or the USA. One of his six siblings died at age 25 with an unknown progressive lung ailment.

Physical examination was notable for a thin male, BP=110/75, HR=104, respiratory rate = 22, oxygen saturation = 96% at rest; chest with diminished breath sounds and a prolonged expiratory phase, slightly elevated jugular venous pressure, midline apex beat (point of maximal impulse [PMI], scaphoid abdomen, no hepatomegaly, but with a trace of pedal oedema. His haematocrit was 45% and other laboratory tests were normal.

Chest radiograph shows flat diaphragm with increased radiolucency at the lung bases.

Lung function tests	Measured	% Predicted
FEV_1 (L)	0.80	20
FVC (L)	3.0	60
FEV_1/FVC	0.27	33
TLC (L)	8.1	120
$D_L co$ (mL/min/mmHg)	14	45

Questions
1 What would you expect the patient's FRC and RV to be?
2 Why is the cardiac PMI shifted to the midline?
3 Why is the FVC low?
4 Why is the $D_L\mathrm{co}$ low?

5 What will happen to the patient's oxygenation with exercise? Why?
6 Why is the patient's jugular venous pressure elevated?
7 What are the most likely diagnosis and pathophysiology of his disease?

Case 3: Restrictive ventilatory defect

Two 60-year-old patients are being evaluated for dyspnoea. On examination, both patients have an oxygen saturation of 88%, small lung volumes to percussion and normal cardiac examinations. Patient A has diffuse bilateral inspiratory crackles and digital clubbing. Patient B has clear lungs and difficulty in rising from his chair and raising his hands over his head.

Questions

1 What patterns of abnormalities do these patients exhibit?
2 Based on the lung function results, what is the most likely pathophysiology explaining each patient's symptoms?
3 What is the likely explanation for the differences in FRC and RV between the two patients?
4 What is the differential diagnosis for Patient A?
5 What is the differential diagnosis for Patient B?
6 Both patients have hypoxemia. Which patient is more likely to have hypercapnia?

Lung function tests	Patient A		Patient B	
	Measured	% Predicted	Measured	% Predicted
FEV$_1$ (L)	1.1	26	1.1	26
FVC (L)	1.3	26	1.3	26
FEV$_1$/FVC	0.80	100	0.80	100
TLC (L)	3.0	43	3.8	54
FRC (L)	2.0	54	3.1	87
RV (L)	1.7	65	2.5	120
$D_L\mathrm{co}$ (mL/min/mmHg)	18	50	36	100

Case 4: Haemoptysis

A 31-year-old married Vietnamese woman presented to the emergency room following an episode of haemoptysis in which she had expectorated 250 mL of fresh red blood. Nasopharyngeal examination by the ENT surgeons was normal, and a chest radiograph (Fig. 40) in casualty was unhelpful, although bronchial wall thickening was noted behind the heart (arrow). There was no further bleeding, and she was discharged with an outpatient appointment. Over the next few days, she continued to expectorate small clots of blood mixed with discoloured phlegm.

At her outpatient appointment, she reported a 10-year history of recurrent, intermittent haemoptysis in which she had expectorated small quantities of fresh red blood, sometimes mixed with bronchial secretions. She had been investigated by several doctors, but chest radiographs were normal, and she had been reassured that the bleeding was from the upper respiratory tract. For the 6 months before her presentation to casualty, she had coughed up small quantities of blood every 2–3 weeks (<50 mL), but there was no associated fever, wheeze or breathlessness on these occasions. Two weeks before presentation to the emergency room, she developed a cough productive of purulent sputum and night-time sweating. As a child, she had suffered with whooping cough, but there was no other past medical history of serious chest illness or tuberculosis. She was a non-smoker.

Examination was normal. She did not have finger clubbing, anaemia, cyanosis or lymphadenopathy. Chest examination was unremarkable. The breath sounds were vesicular, and there were no crackles or wheezes. Routine blood tests, including an ESR and C-reactive protein and sputum microbiology including examination for tuberculosis, were normal. The grade 1 Heaf test was consistent with immunity to tuberculosis.

Questions

1 What are the commonest causes of haemoptysis, and from which circulation does bleeding occur?
2 Is haemoptysis life-threatening, and how is the severity of bleeding classified?
3 What are the clinical features that may help establish the diagnosis? What is the most likely cause in this case?
4 What investigations would you perform to establish the diagnosis in this case?
5 What is bronchiectasis, and what causes it?
6 How should a large haemoptysis be managed?

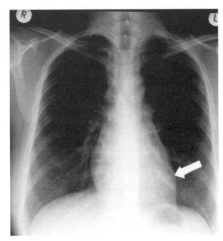

Fig. 40 Chest radiograph.

41 Case studies: answers

Case 1: Asthma

1 For males, peak flow should be no more than 100 L/min below the predicted; Tom's peak flow is therefore within the normal range for his age and size. The most useful value to compare it with would be his own best peak flow rate.

2 All of these should be normal. Asthma, especially in the young, is reversible, and usually between attacks patients have normal airway resistance, compliance, lung volumes and blood gases. Peak flow and auscultation (but see note in answer 9) suggest little evidence of airway obstruction today.

3 Simple observations that can be made in these circumstances:
• How breathless is he? Inability to talk in complete sentences is an indication of a severe attack.
• Respiratory rate (>25 breaths per minute suggests a severe attack).
• Cyanosis (very severe attack).
• Pulse rate (>110 beats per minute suggests a severe attack).
• If he has his peak flow meter with him a value <50% of his best or predicted suggests severe attack.
Even in the absence of the above signs of a severe attack, it is important to monitor the response to treatment to ensure that improvement rather than deterioration is occurring. He should use a short-acting β_2-adrenoreceptor agonist (salbutamol), which relaxes bronchial smooth muscle (see Chapter 22).

4 He now has definite bronchoconstriction; we would expect both peak flow and FEV_1/FVC to be reduced. In this mild attack, he would probably be able to exhale completely, so FRC is likely to be normal. There is at present no reason why lung compliance should be altered. Although he will be working harder than normal, he should be achieving a normal alveolar ventilation and his blood gases should be normal. A reduced arterial P_{CO_2} may be caused by anxiety and consequent hyperventilation.

5 Expiratory rhonchi (musical sounds caused by vibration of the sides of collapsing airways).

6 The broken sentences, use of accessory muscles, high heart and respiratory rate are all important. The peak flow is only about 40% of his best value.

7 This is clearly a severe asthma attack, and airway resistance would be greatly increased. It is likely that air trapping would occur, as initially expiration is affected more than inspiration. As expiration is slowed, the subject may be forced to breathe in before the last breath has been fully exhaled, or air may be trapped behind collapsed airways. This would lead to a raised FRC. The volume/pressure curve flattens as TLC is approached, i.e. compliance is reduced. Consequently, with this severity of attack, the work of breathing is increased not only because of increased work against airway resistance, but because of increased elastic resistance. In addition, with increased FRC, the inspiratory muscles may not be at their optimum working length and hence efficiency is impaired. Some ventilation–perfusion mismatching would be expected, as bronchoconstriction and inflammation will result in underventilation of some regions, and with the resulting shunt effect there is likely to be some degree of arterial hypoxia. Increased total ventilation will usually lower the P_{CO_2}, resulting in a final blood gas picture of low P_{O_2} and low P_{CO_2}.

8 The cyanosis indicates severe hypoxia, and is probably responsible for his confused mental state. The inability to talk and produce a peak flow reading are also signs of life-threatening asthma. The disappearance of rhonchi is consistent with very poor air movement. Rhonchi are a characteristic feature of airway obstruction, but they are not a reliable indicator of severity. In life-threatening asthma, the normal vesicular breath sounds are also absent. A silent chest in an asthma attack is an ominous sign.

9 The low P_aO_2 is caused by ventilation–perfusion mismatching. Hypoxia is what kills in severe asthma, so it is appropriate to give high inspired oxygen, which should significantly raise alveolar oxygen tension in poorly ventilated regions of his lung, and so improve arterial oxygenation. In this patient, there is no need to worry about ventilatory drive, so as high as possible is the correct emergency treatment. With a face mask, the maximum achievable is ~60%. Although a P_{CO_2} of 5.5 kPa would usually be considered 'normal', in the presence of severe hypoxia it should be regarded as worrying. With this degree of hypoxia, the drive to breathing should be increased, with increased ventilation and low P_{CO_2}. Here the failure to raise ventilation appropriately is likely to indicate exhaustion. The patient may deteriorate rapidly—a further fall in ventilation will worsen hypoxia, and this may be fatal. In the presence of significant hypoxia, a 'normal' or high arterial P_{CO_2} should be regarded as a serious finding.

Case 2: Severe breathlessness

1 The obstructive ventilatory defect (low ratio of FEV_1/FVC) coupled with a reduced diffusing capacity for carbon monoxide would suggest emphysema. Emphysema is characterized by a reduction in lung elastic recoil, increased lung compliance and floppy airways. Therefore, FRC and RV are both likely to be elevated.

2 The hyperinflation of the lung and the increase in FRC pulls the apex of the heart caudally and to the middle. This can be seen radiographically as a small midline heart. The ECG will show low voltage due to the increased amount of air between the heart and the chest wall, with an axis close to 90°. For a similar reason, the apex beat may be quiet.

3 The FVC is low because the RV is high. Airways close prematurely in emphysema, which increases RV. Furthermore, because of the marked decrease in maximal expiratory flow rate due to the decreased lung elastic recoil, patients' spirometry traces may not plateau, indicating that the lung was still emptying at very low flow rates when the FVC manoeuvre was terminated.

4 Diffusing capacity is influenced by the alveolar–capillary surface

area for gas exchange. Emphysema is characterized by a loss of the alveolar–capillary units that are utilized for diffusion. There need not be a defect in transfer of gas from the alveolus to the capillary to reduce the D_LCO; a reduction in surface area is adequate to cause abnormality.

5 With exercise, the patient's oxygen saturation will fall because of the diffusion defect. With this magnitude of diffusion defect, the red cells have adequate time to equilibrate with alveolar oxygen as they traverse the alveolar–capillary membrane. However, during exercise, when cardiac output rises, red cells traverse the alveolar–capillary membrane at rest more quickly and do not equilibrate with alveolar oxygen tension at the end-capillary segment. This results in deoxygenated blood entering the systemic circulation when cardiac output is increased. This exercise-induced desaturation will be accentuated when alveolar oxygen is reduced, such as at high altitude. The threshold for significant oxygen desaturation with exercise is approximately D_LCO < 50% predicted.

6 The patient probably has a component of pulmonary hypertension due to the emphysema. The loss of capillary units raises pulmonary vascular resistance and increases right heart work.

Any degree of hypoxaemia during exercise will exacerbate the pulmonary hypertension by superimposing hypoxic pulmonary vasoconstriction on the already increased resistance.

7 The presence of early-onset emphysema, the family history and the history of cigarette smoking make the diagnosis of α_1-antitrypsin (AAT) deficiency most likely. He probably has the homozygous ZZ genotype that causes a marked reduction of AAT levels to <15% normal. The radiograph is consistent with panacinar emphysema and alveolar destruction predominantly at the bases. The lung destruction is due to release of proteolytic enzymes from neutrophils and other inflammatory cells in response to environmental stimuli. These enzymes are normally neutralized by the antiproteases in the lung to prevent lung destruction in the presence of mild inflammatory stimuli. In AAT deficiency, the proteases are not neutralized, and induce panacinar emphysema under 'normal' circumstances. Cigarette smoking induces a neutrophilic response in the lung that accelerates the decline of lung function in AAT deficiency. Intravenous replacement of AAT in patients with reduced lung function may slow the decline in FEV_1.

Case 3: Restrictive ventilatory defect

1 Both patients have restrictive ventilatory defects based on the reduced TLC. FEV_1 and FVC are reduced proportionally, so the FEV_1/FVC is normal; therefore there is no obstructive ventilatory defect. Patient A has reduced D_LCO, signifying a gas transfer defect.

2 Restrictive ventilatory defects may be due to stiff lungs, stiff chest wall, or weak respiratory muscles. Diseases causing stiff lungs will reduce all lung volumes/capacities simultaneously, including TLC, FRC, and RV. Most parenchymal lung diseases will also cause a reduced D_LCO, whereas chest wall disease and respiratory muscle disease will not. An increased RV is also not compatible with stiff lungs. Thus, Patient A seems to have a problem with stiff lungs. The relatively normal FRC and D_LCO in Patient B suggest that the lungs and chest wall are normal. Either a stiff chest wall or weak muscles may cause an increased RV. Patient B's lung function and difficulty in rising out of a chair and raising his arms suggest a muscle disease. Diseases causing weak respiratory muscles will reduce TLC, because the patient cannot inspire deeply.

3 The FRC is determined by the balance between the inward pull of the lung elastic recoil pressure and the outward pull of the chest wall. Therefore, FRC will be reduced if either the net lung recoil pressure increases (due to stiff, low-compliance lungs), or if the net outward pull of the chest wall decreases (for example when scarring of the chest wall produces an added inward recoiling force). Since FRC is determined by the balance between two opposing static forces, respiratory muscle weakness should not influence FRC. However, in clinical practice, patients with respiratory muscle weakness often have a slightly reduced FRC. The mechanism for this finding is probably related to the lack of deep breaths or sighs causing microatelectasis that will increase lung recoil and decrease compliance.

RV is the amount of gas remaining in the lung at the end of maximal expiration. In adults, RV is determined by airway collapse at low lung volumes. However, this presupposes adequate expiratory muscle strength to actively lower lung volume below FRC (which can be reached from TLC passively). Patient A has normal muscle strength and airways that resist collapse due to the parenchymal lung disease, resulting in a reduced RV. Patient B has weak expiratory muscles, resulting in an elevated RV.

4 The differential diagnosis is long, and includes the disorders discussed in Chapter 27. Briefly, these would include occupational/environmental disorders, connective tissue/autoimmune diseases, drug/treatment-induced diseases, primary lung disorders or idiopathic disorders. Idiopathic pulmonary fibrosis or cryptogenic fibrosing alveolitis is likely in a 60-year-old with lung crackles, clubbing, no significant past history, no signs or symptoms of extrapulmonary disease, and the lung function shown for Patient A.

5 Respiratory muscle weakness may be due to a variety of neuromuscular diseases that can involve the spinal cord, motor nerves, neuromuscular junction or skeletal muscles:

• Spinal cord: tumour, syringomyelia, polio, amyotrophic lateral sclerosis, tetanus.

• Motor nerves: brachial/phrenic nerve neuritis, trauma.

• Neuromuscular junction: myasthenia gravis, botulism, organophosphate poisoning.

• Skeletal muscle: muscular dystrophy, myositis, mitochondrial disease, myopathy (nutritional, drug, metabolic, inherited).

6 Hypoxaemia in interstitial lung diseases is usually due to ventilation–perfusion mismatching. Patient A likely has hypocapnia, because patients with interstitial lung disease tend to hyperventilate in response to stiff lungs and hypoxia. This will lower arterial carbon dioxide tension. In contrast, Patient B likely has hypoxaemia due to alveolar hypoventilation, and is therefore hypercapnic. Patient B is also more likely to develop acute respiratory failure with the limited ventilatory reserve due to the muscle weakness.

Case 4: Haemoptysis

1 The table below illustrates that most cases of haemoptysis are due to infection (~80%) — including tuberculosis, pneumonia, lung abscess and bronchiectasis. Only a minority are due to malignancy (~20%). Pulmonary embolism and trauma are other potentially important causes. The bronchial (rather than the pulmonary) circulation is the usual source of bleeding.

2 Approximately 35–40% of cases of haemoptysis are classified as trivial (flecks of blood in sputum), 45–50% as moderate (<500 mL or 0.5–2 cups daily) and only 10–20% as massive (>500 mL or more than 2 cups of blood daily). Mortality is directly related to the rate and volume of blood loss and the underlying pathology. In patients expectorating >500 mL of blood within a 4-h period, the mortality is ~70%, compared to 5% in patients expectorating the same quantity over 16–48 h. Death results from asphyxia, caused by flooding of the alveoli and only rarely from circulatory collapse.

3 A good history is essential, and may indicate the cause of haemoptysis. The characteristic clinical picture of diseases like tuberculosis, bronchiectasis and bronchogenic carcinoma may direct subsequent investigation and management. Chest examination may reveal localized crepitations or consolidation but widespread soiling of the tracheobronchial tree with blood (due to coughing), often results in diffuse clinical signs. Examination of expectorated blood may provide clues. Food particles suggest the possibility of haematemesis, but blood in the nasogastric aspirate does not differentiate between haematemesis and haemoptysis, as coughed-up blood is often swallowed. Purulent material in the sputum may indicate bronchiectasis or a lung abscess. Associated haematuria raises the

Infective (~80%)	Malignant (~20%)	Other
Tuberculosis	Lung cancer	Pulmonary infarction
Pneumonia	Metastatic cancer	Adenoma
Lung abscess	Lymphoma	Traumatic
Bronchiectasis		Alveolar haemorrhage
Aspergillus		Vasculitis

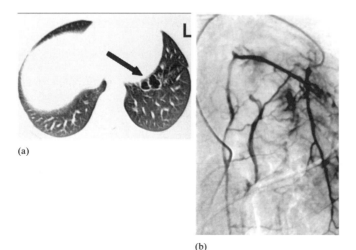

(a)

(b)

Fig. 41 (a) CT scan, (b) bronchial arteriography.

possibility of an alveolar haemorrhage syndrome. In this case, the age of the patient, the long history of minor haemoptysis and the symptoms of purulent sputum and night-time fever suggest a diagnosis of **bronchiectasis**, although other potential causes include recurrent pulmonary emboli, vasculitis and a benign adenoma.

4 Routine blood tests (white cell count raised in infection), including ESR (raised in vasculitis) and C-reactive protein (raised in infection). Specialist blood tests (D-dimers for pulmonary emboli, *Aspergillus* precipitans, vasculitis screen) may be required. Sputum microbiology may isolate infective organisms (pneumonia, abscess, *Aspergillus*) or acid-fast bacilli (tuberculosis). A screening Heaf test may detect tuberculosis. Chest radiography should be obtained in all patients. It may provide important diagnostic information including evidence of a mass, cavity, or abscess. CT scans with contrast may detect the site of bleeding, tumours, vascular malformations and other structural abnormalities. In this case, the CT scan demonstrated a grossly dilated bronchus (>10 mm) consistent with bronchiectasis in the anteromedial segment of the left lower lobe (Fig. 41a). Bronchoscopy is often required to detect endobronchial lesions and inhaled objects (e.g. tooth). Combinations of bronchoscopy and CT scanning have the highest diagnostic yield. Bronchial arteriography may be required to detect the site of bleeding (Fig. 41b).

5 Bronchiectasis is described in Chapter 30.

6 The key aspects of management of massive haemoptysis are to maintain a patent airway and oxygenation (oxygen therapy). Asphyxia (not bleeding) is the greatest immediate risk to the patient. Promote drainage of blood and prevent alveolar 'soiling' by positioning the patient slightly head down in the lateral decubitus position, with the 'presumed' bleeding side down. Determine the cause, site and severity of the bleeding (as above): haematemesis and upper airways bleeding (e.g. nose) may be confused with haemoptysis. Treatment of the underlying cause is essential if the haemoptysis is to be controlled (antibiotics for pneumonia or a lung abscess). Avoid excessive chest manipulation, including physiotherapy, as this may increase or restart bleeding. Cough suppression with codeine 30–60 mg every 6 h may be helpful. Institute appropriate antibiotics and bronchodilators.

Immediate control of haemoptysis is achieved at bronchoscopy by directing boluses of iced saline with epinephrine (10 mL; 1 : 10 000 dilution) at the bleeding site.

Bronchial angiography and embolization are the established therapeutic techniques for the initial control of haemoptysis. This procedure is initially successful in 70–100% of cases. The best results are described in patients with dilated bronchial arteries (e.g. bronchiectasis). Rebleeding often occurs (~40%), and infarction of the anterior spinal artery with paraplegia is reported (~5%). Most studies agree that surgical therapy is associated with the best long-term outcomes for isolated lesions. Primary medical management may be mandatory because bleeding cannot be localized (widespread *Aspergillus* infection) or is not amenable to surgical resection of a pulmonary segment. In other patients, surgery will be contraindicated because of end-stage lung disease (FEV_1 <40% predicted), poor cardiac reserve, unresectable cancer, or severe bleeding diathesis.

Final diagnosis: bronchiectasis of the anteromedial segment of the left lower lobe.

Index